INTERNATIONAL PHARMACY GRADUATES' ROADMAP

YOUR GUIDE TO LICENSURE AND RESIDENCY IN THE UNITED STATES

DANYA ALMHEIRI

ISBN: 978-9948687894 (paperback)

ISBN: 978-9948691488 (eBook)

Veridian House FZE LLC, Sharjah, United Arab Emirates

PREFACE

I wrote this book to provide clarity on a path that is often unclear.

As a pharmacist trained outside the US, I spent years navigating a complex system that often isn't fully explained, including licensure challenges, immigration procedures, unpaid internships, and the pharmacy residency match. Each mistake cost me time, money, and progress. I hope this book will help you avoid those same pitfalls so you can have a better and more informed start.

What you're holding is a practical roadmap rooted in real experience, not just theory. This guide aims to provide you with the essential knowledge and strategies to confidently and effectively handle the US licensure and residency procedures.

It is designed to be action oriented, with step-by-step strategies organized by phases, from preparing in your home country to entering the US system, completing your internship, and preparing for residency. It offers flexibility suited for those self-navigating or enrolled in a bridging program. Throughout, you'll find abbreviations, timelines, and real-world examples to ground each section.

However, this isn't a book you can skim or read out of order.

The process of US licensure and residency is much more complicated than can be covered in a single chapter. Every step you take impacts what happens next. Immigration, licensing, and training are closely interconnected, and understanding one phase without the others can result in costly delays or missed opportunities. Each chapter builds on the previous one. To ensure you have a comprehensive understanding of how to navigate this system strategically, it's essential to read the entire book, as it will empower you with the knowledge and insights needed to make informed decisions and plan your next steps effectively.

By the end, you'll not only understand the process but also learn how to navigate it intentionally. Covering topics from exams and documentation to state board regulations, immigration pathways, and residency challenges, this roadmap is designed to help you begin more strategically, plan effectively, and sidestep common delays many capable pharmacists face.

This isn't about taking shortcuts; it's about providing clear direction.

Let's begin.

ABBREVIATION

Abbr	Full Term
ACPE	Accreditation Council for Pharmacy Education
ASHP	American Society of Health-System Pharmacists
ATT	Authorization to Test
BOP	Board of Pharmacy
CAPPS	Certificate of Advanced Pharmacy Practice Studies
CPJE	California Practice Standards and Jurisprudence Examination
CV	Curriculum Vitae
EAD	Employment Authorization Document
ECE	Educational Credential Evaluators
ETS	Educational Testing Service
F-1	Student Visa Classification
FIC	FPGEE Identification Card
FPGEC	Foreign Pharmacy Graduate Examination Certificate
FPGEE	Foreign Pharmacy Graduate Equivalency Examination
H-1B	Temporary Work Visa for Specialty Occupations
ID	Identification Document
LAU	Lebanese American University
MCPHS	Massachusetts College of Pharmacy and Health Sciences
MPJE	Multistate Pharmacy Jurisprudence Examination
MUSC	Medical University of South Carolina
NABP	National Association of Boards of Pharmacy
NAPLEX	North American Pharmacist Licensure Examination
NMS	National Matching Services
OPT	Optional Practical Training
PGY-1	Postgraduate Year One Pharmacy Residency
PGY-2	Postgraduate Year Two Pharmacy Residency
PhORCAS	Pharmacy Online Residency Centralized Application Service
TOEFL	Test of English as a Foreign Language
USCIS	US Citizenship and Immigration Services

TABLE OF CONTENTS

Chapter 1 | 1
Three Paths to Becoming a US Licensed Pharmacist

Chapter 2 | 17
Roadmap to U.S. Licensure and Residency (Path 2 & 3)

Chapter 3 | 29
The Foundation: Phase One

Chapter 4 | 45
Transition: Phase Two

Chapter 5 | 65
Advancement: Phase Three

Chapter 6 | 87
Match Rates, Trends, and Strategic Insight

CHAPTER 1

THREE PATHS TO BECOMING A US LICENSED PHARMACIST

Section 1: The US Licensure Landscape

The United States does not have a centralized licensing system for pharmacists; instead, licensing is governed by a combination of national coordination and individual state authorities. It is crucial to understand the distinction between these levels from the outset. At the national level, the primary governing organization is the National Association of Boards of Pharmacy (NABP). This organization does not issue licenses but oversees the key components of the licensure process for both US-trained and foreign-trained pharmacists.

NABP is responsible for administering several important exams, including the North American Pharmacist Licensure Examination (NAPLEX), the Multistate Pharmacy Jurisprudence Examination (MPJE), and the Foreign Pharmacy Graduate Equivalency Examination (FPGEE). Additionally, it issues the FPGEC Certification, which is a mandatory credential for foreign-trained pharmacists aiming to practice in the US.

Furthermore, NABP sets the minimum required scores for the Test of English as a Foreign Language Internet-based (TOEFL iBT), which is used to assess English language proficiency and is required for international candidates seeking FPGEC certification. However, NABP does not administer the TOEFL exam itself; that responsibility lies with the Educational Testing Service (ETS).

It is important to clarify that NABP's role is purely evaluative and administrative; it does not have the authority to grant licensure to practice pharmacy.

The actual licensing authority resides entirely with each individual state's Board of Pharmacy (BOP). Each state operates under its own specific laws, regulations, and timelines, which makes the licensing process highly variable across the country.

Each state's board of pharmacy determines:

- The required internship hours, typically between 1,500 and 2,080.
- Whether foreign internship experience is accepted.
- If registration as a pharmacy intern is necessary before earning hours.
- The necessary exams:
    - Most states require you to finish your US internship hours before you're eligible to take the NAPLEX.
    - Many also need the MPJE; some use state-specific exams like the California Practice Standards and Jurisprudence Examination (CPJE), Virginia's Pharmacy Law Exam, or Arkansas's Jurisprudence Exam.
- If your license can be transferred to other states later. For instance, California does not participate in NABP's license transfer program and requires the CPJE.

The system is summarized in simple terms. NABP builds the bridge, but each state determines if you can cross it. Licensing in the U.S. is decentralized: national exams and certifications qualify you, but each state board ultimately grants the license. To succeed, you must navigate both systems—following the correct sequence, submitting the right documents, and timing it properly.

Section 2: The Three Entry Paths for Pharmacy Licensure

Becoming a licensed pharmacist in the US does not have a universal entry process, but there are three common, widely recognized routes. All these routes ultimately lead to earning a US pharmacist license. Your chosen route depends on your starting point, existing qualifications, available time and funds, and immigration or professional goals.

Making this decision early helps you plan effectively, avoid setbacks, and save costs. This section explains each pathway clearly and objectively, allowing you to align your choice with your timeline, resources, immigration status/visa, and long-term plans.

1.2.1 US PharmD Degree Pathway

This pathway involves enrolling in a US Doctor of Pharmacy (PharmD) program and offers the most organized, institutionally supported route to US licensure.

Who It's For:

- Individuals without a pharmacy degree, typically international high school or undergraduate students
- Foreign-trained pharmacists whose credentials don't qualify for other options or who are seeking full US academic and clinical integration
- Foreign-trained pharmacists who want to transfer applicable coursework

Key Features:

- **Duration:** Four to six years, depending on the program (shorter for students/graduates transferring their coursework)
- **Cost:** High, with tuition and living expenses totaling $150,000–$200,000+ (less for students/graduates transferring their coursework)
- **Visa:** F-1 student visa, with eligibility for optional practical training (OPT)
- **Support:** Structured with academic advising, internship opportunities, and streamlined eligibility for NAPLEX/MPJE exams
- **Residency Access:** High. PharmD students are integrated into the US system and can compete as traditional applicants.

Coursework Transfer Credits:

Some universities may permit you to transfer applicable coursework from your foreign pharmacy degree. If the curriculum is similar in content and rigor, schools might accept your syllabi for evaluation. This process is akin to transfer student procedures within US institutions. While it won't eliminate the PharmD requirement, it could shorten the program by allowing you to skip certain prerequisite or didactic courses.

Based on my direct experience, certain US pharmacy schools permit foreign pharmacy graduates to transfer their coursework after syllabus assessment. These students are typically admitted into the third year of the PharmD program, needing just one more year of classroom study along with a second year of clinical rotations. This pathway reduces their overall academic time and grants them the official designation of US pharmacy graduates from ACPE-accredited schools, which is a significant advantage when pursuing residency.

This depends entirely on the university's policies and your academic records but can significantly reduce both time and costs if approved.

> **Summary:**
> This path is the most structured yet also the most costly. It provides the clearest route into US residencies and practice but may not be feasible for working pharmacists. This option is ideal for individuals whose pharmacy credentials do not align with US standards, or for international pharmacy graduates who can transfer some of their coursework credits to shorten the PharmD program to two years. For those who choose this route, transfer credits can enhance efficiency if evaluated and accepted early.

1.2.2 FPGEC Pharmacy Bridging Program Pathway

This pathway is designed for pharmacists with a pharmacy degree from outside the US who wish to gain US clinical experience, develop a residency-eligible profile, and prepare for licensure through a structured, university-based program. These programs, often referred to as international pharmacy certificate programs, postgraduate certificates, or bridging pathways, typically include classroom instruction, clinical rotations, and dedicated test preparation support.

Who It's For:

- Foreign-trained pharmacists needing US-based experience, structure, or a visa-sponsored route
- Candidates preparing for FPGEE, TOEFL iBT, and US clinical practice
- Candidates who have completed their FPGEC requirements and ONLY need internship placement
- Those who prefer academic environments over independent navigation

> **Key Features:**
>
> - **Duration:** Usually twelve to twenty-four months
> - **Cost:** Moderate to high ($40,000–$80,000, depending on the program and location)
> - **Visa:** F-1 student visa, often accompanied by OPT work authorization afterward
> - **Support:** Moderate to high. Most programs help with FPGEE and TOEFL prep, provide access to rotation sites, and guide on NAPLEX/MPJE timelines.
> - **Residency Access:** Medium. Depending on the program structure, university support, clinical rotation site, preceptors, and competitiveness of the application

Academic and Exam Preparation:

A major benefit is preparation for the FPGEE and TOEFL iBT exams, often through dedicated courses, review workshops, and structured timelines to keep you on track.

This support is particularly useful if you're not familiar with US testing expectations, need to improve your language or clinical terminology skills, or require clinical rotation experience to prepare for future residency rotations.

However, these programs do not guarantee a pharmacy residency. Although they can boost your competitiveness through US-based training, preceptor evaluations, and exposure to the residency process, the final decision depends on your complete application, including interview performance, recommendation letters, and your visa or work eligibility at the time of application.

Lastly, if you've already obtained your FPGEC certification, you can request a waiver from the program director to skip the preparatory part of the bridging program, which usually lasts one year. Approved waivers could shorten your overall program duration and tuition from two years to one.

> **Summary:**
>
> This pathway offers a clearer and more organized route for internationally trained pharmacists seeking US licensure. Aimed at individuals requiring academic support and legal entry, these university-based programs typically include preparation for the FPGEE and TOEFL, clinical rotations, and

> assistance with securing a pharmacy internship. Most are available under the F-1 student visa, offering legal status and eligibility for optional practical training (OPT), which is essential for pursuing residency.

1.2.3 Independently Navigating the FPGEC Certification Pathway

This pathway is designed for international pharmacists who want to use their existing pharmacy degree without enrolling in another degree program to pursue US licensure.

This route requires passing the TOEFL iBT, submitting your degree for credential evaluation (ECE), obtaining FPGEC certification through NABP, passing the FPGEE, completing US internship hours, and then passing the NAPLEX and MPJE.

Who It's For:

- Licensed pharmacists with a five-year pharmacy degree from outside the US
- Individuals seeking to avoid repeating their degree and who prefer managing their timeline independently
- Those who already hold a green card
- US citizens by naturalization or family petition
- Individuals sponsored through employment or marriage
- Foreign pharmacists with long-term immigration plans

This path does not offer a built-in visa; applicants must already have or be actively pursuing some form of legal US residency.

This is a critical consideration: Without a legal way to stay in the US to complete the internship and licensure steps, this path becomes difficult or impossible to finish.

Key Features:

- **Duration:** Two to three years on average, depending on planning, internship availability, and exam timelines
- **Cost:** Low to moderate ($15,000–$30,000 total if managed strategically)
- **Visa:** Self-managed, does not include a built-in F-1 or H-1B route. You must already have, or independently obtain, a legal residence status.
- **Support:** Low. You are responsible for planning, paperwork, and selecting states, internships, and sequencing.
- **Residency Access:** Low. Heavily dependent on documentation, legal status, clinical exposure, and timing

Summary:

- The FPGEC route is the most independent and cost-effective, but it requires careful planning, legal foresight, and a clear understanding of your immigration status. It is best suited for pharmacists who already have US legal status or a long-term plan to obtain it.

- Lastly, if you're a foreign-trained pharmacist pursuing the FPGEC certification, your first step in obtaining licensure in the US is through NABP.

Section 3: Which Path Is Right for You?

After reviewing the three entry options, the choice is personal: Which one genuinely suits you, not just on paper but in real life? There's no flawless route. Instead, choose the path that matches your existing documents, your legal status (or potential status), your available funding and time, the support level you need, and your long-term goals, whether that's US residency, permanent employment, or returning home (see appendix A).

For those who are not a green card holder or have no immigration plan, avoid selecting a route solely based on time or cost. The deciding factor is your legal status. Without the appropriate visa or immigration strategy, even the cheapest or most adaptable route can fail partway. Begin by confirming how you can legally remain, study, and work in the US. This crucial point narrows your options more effectively than any checklist.

1.3.1 Strategic Questions to Help Choose Your Path

If you're reading this, you probably aim to obtain pharmacy licensure and residency in the US. Your focus is on using your time, resources, and legal options effectively to achieve this goal in the most strategic and feasible manner. Before you begin planning, pause for a moment to reflect.

Let's go through a few questions. They aren't a test but are designed to clear up confusion and prevent false starts. Don't choose a course of action simply because it appears easiest or most popular. Select based on what's realistic for your situation—and what offers the best chance of completing it, not just starting. If you answer "yes" to most questions below, that path might be the best fit for you.

Path 1: US PharmD

- Are you just starting your education and do not yet hold a pharmacy degree?
- Does your pharmacy degree fulfill NABP's minimum educational requirements for US licensure? If no, this is your only option. If yes,
    - Do you think your previous coursework and academic record are strong enough for your syllabi to be accepted for advanced placement or course waivers?
    - Do you have access to funding or a scholarship that can cover over $150K for tuitioen and living expenses?
    - Do you want to fully immerse yourself in the US academic and clinical environment from the beginning?
    - Are you looking for a supportive environment with built-in academic advisors, rotations, and internships?

Path 2: FPGEC Bridging Certificate Program

- Do you already possess a pharmacy degree from outside the US?
- Does your pharmacy degree fulfill NABP's minimum educational requirements for US licensure?
- Are you seeking organized support and guidance to prepare for the FPGEE and TOEFL iBT at a US university?
- Would you prefer guaranteed access to rotations at US hospitals rather than searching for internships independently?
- Are you comfortable spending $40K–$80K on a one- to two-year program without a guaranteed residency?

Path 3: Independent FPGEC Path

- Do you hold a five-year pharmacy degree and an active license in your home country?
- Does your pharmacy degree fulfill NABP's minimum educational requirements for US licensure?
- Do you want to avoid repeating your degree and save costs?
- Are you self-motivated and capable of managing paperwork, deadlines, and legal procedures independently?

- Do you have or plan to obtain legal status in the US, such as a green card or another immigration route?

Section 4: What Is the Focus of This Book?

This book reviews the FPGEC certification process, crucial for international pharmacists aiming to obtain licensure in the US with their current degrees and desiring to strengthen their applications for pharmacy residency programs. Whether you follow a bridging program (path two) or an independent route (path three), the core steps remain the same: verifying credentials, meeting English standards, passing the FPGEE, completing US internship hours, and ultimately passing the NAPLEX and MPJE exams. The main difference lies in the level of support available. Bridging programs often provide guidance, exam preparation, and legal and transition support, whereas independent candidates handle all requirements themselves, including documentation, timelines, internships, and legal aspects. This guide caters to pharmacists pursuing either path, as both are striving for FPGEC certification and US licensure. I highlight the main activities of both pathways because they are less documented and often misunderstood and carry serious consequences if overlooked. Whether with institutional help or on your own, this book serves as your essential roadmap.

CHAPTER 2

ROADMAP TO U.S. LICENSURE AND RESIDENCY (PATH 2 & 3)

With a strong understanding of U.S. licensure pathways for international pharmacy graduates, the next step is to plan your journey from your home country to a pharmacy residency in the United States, whether through Path 2 (bridging programs) or Path 3 (self-directed FPGEC certification). Success depends on coordinating exam schedules, applications, and immigration processes with internships and residencies. Viewing these steps as a unified plan enables you to build a compliant and competitive profile aligned with U.S. standards, thereby increasing your chances of securing a residency.

Section 1: US Pharmacy Residency Roadmap: A Three-Phase Commitment for International Pharmacists

The roadmap begins with the NABP's basic requirements: having a five-year pharmacy degree (like a Bachelor of Pharmacy or PharmD) and keeping an active license in the country where you studied. Each phase then details the key requirements, timelines, and decisions affecting your eligibility, costs, and competitiveness. This structured method enhances your credentials and greatly improves your chances of securing a U.S. pharmacy residency.

2.1.1 Phase 1: The Foundation — While You're Still in Your Country

The initial step for every competitive candidate is establishing a solid foundation before entering the US system. This preparatory phase emphasizes qualification, documentation, and strategy. It involves positioning yourself strategically by organizing documents, verifying credentials, choosing your target state in the US, and preparing for the FPGEE and TOEFL—all while still in your home country.

Key Objectives:

- Verify your eligibility.
- Start the FPGEC application process.
- Understand and reassess your strategy to secure legal status, enabling you to enter, stay, and work in the US throughout your internship and post-licensure period.

Action Steps:

- Graduate from an accredited pharmacy program that meets NABP's minimum education standards, usually a five-year program. Shorter programs may disqualify you from FPGEC certification unless supplemented by bridging degrees through transferring your course-work to a US PharmD program.
- You need to hold an active pharmacist license from the country where you obtained your pharmacy degree, as mandated by NABP for FPGEC eligibility. If you do not meet this requirement, don't worry; we will discuss strategic solutions in a later chapter.
- Take the TOEFL iBT exam as proof of English proficiency. It must be taken in the US, Canada, or an NABP-recognized country. You can attempt a practice test or local sitting first to assess readiness. For additional information, consistently consult the latest edition of the FPGEC Candidate Application Bulletin available on the NABP website.

- Meet the required TOEFL iBT scores per section, not as an average.
- Start your FPGEC application with NABP by collecting and submitting documents to educational credential evaluators (ECE) for degree evaluation.
- Once approved, register for the FPGEE and prepare for the exam; preparation typically takes three to six months based on your background.
- Select your target state for licensure early. This decision is strategic, not just administrative, because each state has different rules regarding internship hours, intern licensure applications, acceptance of foreign experience, and NAPLEX eligibility.

Choosing the wrong state can push back your timeline by over a year. Some boards may take months to respond or might reject applicants due to administrative technicalities. Others are quicker, more adaptable, or more welcoming to foreign-trained applicants. Your choice of state has a significant impact on your timeline, expenses, internship opportunities, and future job prospects. Make your decision based on your long-term goals rather than initial convenience.

2.1.2 Phase 2: Transition — Moving to the US for Internship and Licensure, and Preparing for Residency

This is the implementation phase, which involves relocating to the US, starting your internship, and completing licensure requirements. Many applicants face difficulties here, not due to unclear steps, but because of issues with legal status, timing, and coordination. Two main legal entry options exist:

- Via education: enrolling in a US-based certificate or bridging program (typically under an F-1 visa)
- Via independent entry: using a green card, a dependent visa, or other legal stay allowing internship completion

Key Objectives:

- Relocate with a valid legal status.
- Register and obtain your intern license through the BOP.
- Complete the required internship hours.
- Pass the licensure exams (NAPLEX and MPJE).

Action Steps:

- Secure legal entry into the US.
- If joining a bridging program, typically obtain an F-1 visa.
- If entering independently, ensure you have another legal status such as a green card or dependent visa.
- Obtain your intern license by applying to your state board, noting that requirements vary—some may ask for fingerprints, interviews, or notarized documents. The processing time can range from weeks to months, so plan ahead.
- Start accruing internship hours: Most states require 1,500–2,080 supervised hours under a licensed pharmacist. These hours must be documented and submitted for review. They can often be completed at retail

chains, hospitals, or community pharmacies, but a licensed pharmacist is required.

- Prepare for and pass the NAPLEX, which is a clinical competency exam that often requires candidates to study for three to five months.
- Also prepare for and pass the MPJE or the state-specific law exam, which tests your knowledge of pharmacy regulations. Since the exam is state-specific, moving to a new state might require retaking it.

2.1.3 Phase 3: Advancement — Residency and Postgraduate Status

This is the phase where candidates move from intern to professional, setting themselves up for postgraduate training and long-term career stability. This phase is competitive and time sensitive and depends on immigration status.

Key Objectives:

- Match into a PGY-1 residency.
- Secure work authorization.
- Complete licensure requirements if not already achieved in the second phase.

You can begin applying for PGY-1 residency programs before passing the NAPLEX and MPJE exams. However, keep in mind that once your residency begins, you'll have only ninety days to successfully complete both exams. While this is a common route taken by many residents, I strongly advise completing both exams before starting your PGY-1, if possible. The first ninety days of residency are extremely demanding—with heavy clinical workloads, onboarding, and numerous assignments—leaving little time or mental space for board exam preparation.

Action Steps:

- Apply for PGY-1 during the residency match cycle, meeting all program-specific requirements (clinical experience, CV, letters of recommendation, etc.).
- Build a comprehensive application: US internship hours, clinical experience, letters of recommendation, a compelling personal statement and CV, and relevant research or leadership experience if applicable. Also, understand your visa and work status.
- At this phase, your immigration/work status is critical:
    - If you're still under F-1 status, apply for optional practical training (OPT) to gain temporary work authorization.
    - Some employers might sponsor you for an H-1B visa during or after your residency, mostly in PGY-2.
    - If eligible, pursuing or having a green card may simplify long-term employment options and increase program competitiveness.

2.1.4 Common Pitfalls in the FPGEC Process

The most common obstacle for international applicants isn't lack of intelligence, motivation, or qualifications. It's misalignment between timelines and documentation, immigration status and licensure requirements, and effort and strategy. Many start this journey thinking that completing key steps such as passing the TOEFL or submitting the FPGEC application means they're progressing. However, licensure and residency in the US are complex systems with interconnected layers and hidden dependencies, not simple checklists.

Applicants often get derailed not by failing exams but by mistakes like submitting documents to the wrong office, sending TOEFL scores before opening an NABP account, selecting the wrong state based on a forum comment, or applying for internships without legal work authorization. These errors can be fixed if you recognize them early, but most people don't realize they're happening until it's too late.

Common Administrative and Documentation Errors

- Submitting incomplete or unsealed documents to ECE or NABP
- Sending TOEFL scores prior to opening your NABP account
- Not complying with the two-year documentation window for NABP
- Relying on verbal advice instead of official bulletins

Poor Timing and Sequencing

- Taking TOEFL too late
- Delaying state selection until after FPGEC

2.1.5 Common Pitfalls in the Residency Process

Another common yet often overlooked issue occurs during the transition from internship to residency. Finishing your internship in June leaves almost no time for your state Board of Pharmacy to verify your internship hours; a process that can take several weeks. Without prompt verification, your licensure status might remain incomplete, preventing you from officially starting a residency or delaying your ability to take the NAPLEX and MPJE within the 90-day window after residency begins. Additionally, delaying your OPT application can create gaps in work authorization; for instance, your OPT might not cover the entire residency period from the end of June through the following July. A similar issue arises when trying to secure a PGY-2 position in a different state without first understanding NABP's license transfer and reciprocity procedures; this can delay or prevent your eligibility if your license isn't recognized on time. Overall, these issues can threaten your residency placement, lead to gaps in legal work status, or force you to take critical exams under severe time constraints.

Incorrect Immigration and Legal Assumptions

- Selecting a state that does not recognize your visa status
- Not applying early enough for intern licensure or OPT
- Expecting to obtain H-1B for the second-year residency
- Ignoring state-specific requirements, such as California's CPJE or NAPLEX retakes

Residency-Readiness Gaps

- Lack of clinical US preceptors, resulting in weak recommendations

- Insufficient inpatient rotations or absence of PGY-1-aligned clinical experiences
- Failure to verify that your OPT aligns with your residency state's requirements
- Assuming PGY-2 acceptance will automatically follow PGY-1

2.1.6 Strategic Checklist to Assess Your Readiness

If you've followed the roadmap so far, you likely have a clearer understanding of the requirements, challenges, and timelines ahead. However, understanding the process doesn't mean you're ready to start. This checklist is designed to help you pause, assess your readiness, and identify any missing components before proceeding with confidence.

Readiness Checklist (see appendix B)

- I am fully aware of my visa status or have a realistic plan to obtain legal authorization for internship and residency.
- I have achieved the required TOEFL iBT scores, and they are still valid.
- I know which documents must be sent directly from my university or health authority to NABP or ECE.
- I have collected, translated, and sealed the necessary documents (transcripts, licenses, letters).
- I have started preparing for the FPGEE or have a structured study plan in place.
- I have identified the US state I will target for licensure and residency, based on realistic eligibility.

- I understand the state's internship hour requirements and pre-licensure conditions.
- I have a funding plan in place to cover exam fees, relocation, living costs, and any unpaid training phases.
- I have researched pharmacy residency programs that accept international graduates and align with my visa options.
- I have determined which year I will apply for PGY-1 residency, and my timeline aligns with that cycle.

The journey to securing a pharmacy residency in the United States involves three main phases: foundation, transition, and advancement, each with its own goals, milestones, and timelines. This is a broad overview of the entire process to help you see the big picture without turning it into a strict checklist. Every phase includes important decisions, subtle steps, and potential challenges, which will be explained in detail throughout the book so you understand not just what to do, but why and when to do it.

CHAPTER 3

THE FOUNDATION: PHASE ONE

Phase One focuses on building a strong legal, academic, and practical foundation before leaving your home country. Overlooking documents, delaying credentialing, or missing exam deadlines can cause wasted time, additional costs, and reduce your chances of residency later. Following the proper order now provides a strategic edge and ensures smoother progress in upcoming phases.

Section 1: What Is Your Starting Point?

Before you apply to the NABP, it's crucial to establish a clear and well-documented starting point. Many international pharmacists mistakenly jump into exam prep or visa planning without first verifying that their foundational documents and credentials meet US standards . Take a moment to ensure all your documents and credentials align with U.S. standards.

3.1.1 Your Home Country License: An Essential First Credential

You must hold a valid pharmacist license from the country where you earned your degree. This is a mandatory eligibility requirement for the FPGEC certification. Even if you're licensed elsewhere or working in a different country, the NABP focuses on your original country of education.

NABP Requirement: Licensing must be from the same country where your degree was awarded.

This rule ensures your academic training was officially recognized and authorized for practical use by the relevant health authority. Without a license, a degree can raise concerns, indicating it might be incomplete, insufficient, or noncompliant with practice standards.

What if your country doesn't permit licensing due to citizenship, residency, or nationality rules? Let's consider this common scenario.

3.1.2 If Licensing Isn't Possible Where You Earned Your Degree

Some pharmacists may not be able to obtain a license in the country where they graduated. Case example: A non-Jordanian student obtains a PharmD degree from a university in Jordan. However, the Jordanian Ministry of Health exclusively issues pharmacy licenses to Jordanian nationals. As the student does not meet this eligibility criterion, they are consequently unable to obtain a local license, despite fulfilling all academic requirements.

In this case, a specific workaround exists. The student is required to secure an official "To Whom It May Concern" letter from the country where their studies were conducted, in this case Jordan. This document serves as a formal declaration from the health authority affirming the graduate's scientific and professional preparedness, even if they do not fulfill the national licensing conditions. Below is the suggested wording for that letter, which should be requested from the Ministry of Health (or its equivalent):

> *To Whom It May Concern: After reviewing the bachelor's in Pharmacy or PharmD degree conferred upon pharmacist "name of the pharmacist" (nationality) from the University of Jordan (or other university) on "date," please be advised that the abovementioned pharmacist is scientifically and*

technically qualified to practice the profession of pharmacy and can be issued a permanent license to practice the profession of pharmacy in case they obtain the Jordanian nationality (or other nationality). This certificate has been issued to him/her upon the pharmacist's request without any responsibility on the part of the ministry.

Once you obtain this letter:

- Translate the document into English through a certified translation agency.
- Ensure the translator provides a statement such as: I, the undersigned, hereby certify that I am conversant in Arabic (or other language) and English languages, and that the above translation made by me is, to the best of my knowledge and belief, a correct translation of this document from Arabic (or other language) into English.
- Request several copies in sealed, signed, and stamped envelopes from the translation agency.
- Mail this letter through the official mail office within the Ministry of Health (or its equivalent). This is the approach I used myself, and it enhanced the document's credibility and traceability of its origin. If you mail the letter before opening and paying for your NABP account, it might be discarded or lost, it might be discarded or lost. We will review the optimal timing and strategy for opening your NABP account in the next section.

This letter serves as legal confirmation; it does not replace a license but indicates you could obtain one under standard conditions. Therefore, it is acceptable to the NABP. Along with that letter, you must also provide a pharmacy license certificate from the country where you currently practice pharmacy.

3.1.3 Internship Completion Report

Your university may require you to complete a specific number of internship hours as part of your pharmacy program. Keep this certificate as carefully as you do your diploma or transcripts.

Here is the recommended course of action:

- Obtain an official letter or certificate confirming the successful completion of your internship from the relevant authority, be it your university, the school of pharmacy, or the health ministry responsible for pharmacy training.
- Ensure that it includes:
    - The total number of internship hours completed.
    - The specific training period, including start and end dates.
    - The name and license number of your supervising pharmacist, if applicable.
- Have it professionally translated into English by a certified translation agency.
- Prepare multiple sealed, signed, and stamped copies to be kept in envelopes for future use.
- You may need to mail through the official authority mail office if needed.

Although this document is not mandatory for your FPGEC application, it may prove valuable later in the process. For example, this letter may prove beneficial when engaging with US state boards of pharmacy. Certain states permit candidates to submit prior foreign internship experience for evaluation. Although the granting of credit is not guaranteed, submitting this certificate allows you to formally request a reduction in the US internship hours required for licensure, which could significantly reduce your time and effort.

Remember, before departing from the country where you graduated, you must secure multiple copies of these documents in multiple sealed, signed, and stamped envelopes by the authorized translation office, whether for a US pharmacy residency or other reasons, as it is crucial for your next steps in your pharmacy future.

3.1.4 Secure Your English Language Proficiency Exam (TOEFL iBT) Score Prior to Graduation

Before starting your FPGEC certification application, you must demonstrate English proficiency by passing the TOEFL iBT exam. This requirement is mandatory for everyone, regardless of being a native English speaker or having completed pharmacy studies in an English-speaking country. NABP enforces the same standard for all international pharmacy graduates to maintain consistent communication skills across US healthcare settings.

The TOEFL iBT is not just a formality; it is the essential first milestone in your FPGEC journey. Many international pharmacists overlook its importance or delay taking it, not realizing NABP will not begin processing their FPGEC application until it has received passing TOEFL iBT scores from an approved testing center. Therefore, don't start your NABP application until you have passed the TOEFL iBT exam.

To facilitate a smoother progression and reduce potential delays related to the FPGEC application process, I strongly recommend completing the TOEFL iBT prior to graduation. Many students mistakenly believe they must wait until they are fully licensed to initiate any segment of the FPGEC process. However, as NABP does not stipulate that your pharmacy license must be active for a minimum period, you are permitted to complete the TOEFL at an early stage—specifically during your final term of pharmacy studies—and subsequently submit it once your license has been obtained.

It is worth mentioning that the TOEFL iBT can often become a bottleneck early in the application process. It demands dedicated preparation, access to NABP-approved testing centers, and time for official score reporting. Since your TOEFL score remains valid for two years, it's best to take it during your final semester. This way, you will have at least one and a half years of score validity when you're ready to submit your NABP application, saving time and avoiding unnecessary retests.

The passing scores were recently changed to Reading 21, Listening 22, Speaking 25, and Writing 22. For additional information, consistently consult the latest edition of the FPGEC Candidate Application Bulletin available on the NABP website.

The TOEFL iBT test must be taken at an ETS test center that is recognized by NABP. This includes the US, the District of Columbia, Guam, Puerto Rico, the Virgin Islands, and Canada.

Please visit the NABP website for more details. The link is provided in the reference page.

If you are outside these regions, it is advisable to refrain from organizing a brief journey to North America to take the exam until you are assured of your preparedness. Initially, undertake practice under exam conditions within your home country until your scores meet or surpass the established minimum requirements. Only thereafter should you proceed to finalize your travel arrangements. Please note that the examination can only be taken once every three days, and the scores obtained will remain valid for a period of two years.

TOEFL iBT registration permits the transmission of one complimentary score report to NABP. It is prudent to await confirmation. If NABP receives your score before you activate your application, NABP may discard it. However, I suggest forgoing this free opportunity because the expense of sending a new report is cheaper than the $750 you might forfeit if you don't pass the exam within the two-year time frame of your NABP FPGEC application.

Once you pass the TOEFL iBT test in NABP-approved centers, you can proceed to the next step.

Section 2: The General Evaluation Report – ECE

After passing the TOEFL iBT, the next essential step for FPGEC certification is obtaining a general evaluation report from Educational Credential Evaluators (ECE). ECE, authorized by NABP, assesses foreign academic credentials by comparing your pharmacy education against US standards to determine if it meets the basic eligibility for US licensure.

NABP only requires the general evaluation report, not a detailed, course-by-course evaluation. Once finalized, ECE will send this report directly to NABP as part of your FPGEC application.

This report verifies that your pharmacy degree meets NABP's educational requirements and is a key part of your licensure process. You cannot apply for FPGEC certification until your evaluation is complete and received by NABP.

To avoid unnecessary costs and delays, I highly recommend finishing the ECE evaluation before submitting your FPGEC application and paying the $750 fee, but only after you have taken the TOEFL iBT and passed it. This approach prevents submitting an incomplete application and allows time to resolve any issues related to transcripts, degree documents, or translations.

There are a few requirements from NABP regarding how you should mail your credentials to ECE. Both documents should be in a sealed, signed, stamped envelope and must be sent directly from your university or school of pharmacy. Please confirm with your university whether they can send the document directly to ECE online. This is the typical practice in the United Kingdom. However, graduates from Jordan typically need to visit their university registration office to obtain copies of their certificates and transcripts.

If the university registration office can place your document in an envelope and seal it with a stamp and signature, that's acceptable. If not, you should visit the university mail office afterward to request a stamp, signature, and seal on the envelopes before the office sends the documents to the ECE. Please visit the NABP website for more details. The link is provided in the reference page.

If your transcript or degree is in a language other than English, have it translated by a certified translation office. The translator should include a declaration such as: "I, the undersigned, hereby certify that I am conversant in [source language] and English, and that this translation is accurate and complete to the best of my knowledge." Even if your university provides an English version, you might still need to submit both the original document and the certified translation.

The ECE evaluation typically takes six to eight weeks after all documents are received and approved. If your documents are incomplete, incorrect, or not sealed, this will cause delays. Once issued, your general evaluation report remains valid for two years, provided you submit your FPGEC application within that period.

When your ECE general evaluation report is completed, you will be prepared to formally submit your FPGEC application and progress further toward licensure and a pharmacy residency in the United States (see appendix C).

Finally, there's no need to submit your master's or PhD degree to ECE, as the NABP does not require them, and they do not contribute to your FPGEC application.

Section 3: The NABP - FPGEC Application

Once you have successfully passed the TOEFL iBT and obtained your general evaluation report from ECE, you are prepared to submit your application for FPGEC certification through the

National Association of Boards of Pharmacy (NABP). This submission officially activates your file with NABP and marks your formal entry into the US licensure system.

As of June 2025, the application fee is $750 USD, payable via the NABP website (refer to the reference page for direct links). Ensure that you review the most up-to-date fee and application policies outlined in the FPGEC Candidate Application Bulletin prior to submission.

3.3.1 Create Your NABP E-Profile

Prior to submitting your application, you are required to create an NABP e-profile and acquire your NABP ID number. This identifier will be utilized to link all your reports, examinations, and correspondence with NABP. Upon receipt of your NABP ID, log into your TOEFL and ECE profiles and request that both score reports be dispatched directly to NABP. There is no need to employ expedited or rush services; your application cannot advance until all documentation is provided. Standard processing is adequate if submissions are made in a timely manner.

3.3.2 Other Required Documents

Within three months of submitting your online application, NABP requires the following documents. Each must be certified, in English, and meet the exact specifications outlined in the FPGEC Candidate Application Bulletin:

- FPGEC attestation document
- Two passport-size photographs
- Government-issued photo identification (e.g., passport copy)

- Certified pharmacy license

If these items are not submitted within the timeline, your application will be considered incomplete. I can confidently say that my FPGEC evaluation process was smooth, efficient, and issue-free. I believe this outcome was largely due to the specific steps I took during the documentation phase, and I'm sharing them below to help you avoid delays or rejections.

3.3.3 FPGEC Attestation Document, Photograph, and Passport Copy

While NABP permits the attestation document to be signed and stamped by a consular officer, first-class magistrate, or notary public, I strongly recommend having it certified by the US Embassy in your country if possible. Although NABP policy accepts alternative officials (see their website for details), embassy validation adds credibility and reduces the risk of rejection.

Ensure the passport-size photo is partially stamped and that your passport copy is signed and stamped by the US Embassy, if available. If embassy certification isn't feasible, opt for a different authorized translation office than the one used for your educational documents. While not explicitly required, it's advisable to send your documents in a sealed and stamped envelope. The correct NABP mailing address for FPGEC applicants is listed in the FPGEC Candidate Application Bulletin.

3.3.4 Pharmacy License Certification

The pharmacy license must be issued and certified by the relevant government agency in the country of issuance and should be accompanied by an official attestation from the issuing authority, such as the Department of Health.

Your license should be from the institution where you graduated; if not, you can provide the "to whom it may concern" letter discussed in the previous chapter, and include your active license from your current practice location.

The certified license must include the issue date, license number, and any other requirements specified in the FPGEC Candidate Application Bulletin on the NABP website. The document must be placed in a sealed envelope by the issuing agency, with the seal, stamp, or signature overlapping the flap of the envelope. After sealing, you or the issuing agency can send the envelope directly to the NABP.

If the NABP receives only part of your required application documents and the remaining items are not submitted within two years, then:

- All documents previously submitted will be purged (deleted) from your file.
- You will need to restart the entire application process from the beginning, including resubmitting all documentation.

The evaluation process will take approximately eight weeks, as per NABP, but only if your documents are complete and meet all the requirements.

Section 4: The FPGEE Exam

Once your FPGEC application has been reviewed and marked as "accepted" in your NABP account, you become eligible to register for the Foreign Pharmacy Graduate Equivalency

Examination (FPGEE)—the standardized exam that assesses your knowledge of pharmacy practice and science as it relates to US standards.

You can purchase the FPGEE in your NABP account. After payment, Pearson VUE will send you an authorization to test (ATT) letter within two business days, as per NABP guidelines. To register for the exam at your chosen test center, visit the Pearson VUE website and create an account. Please note that the ATT email outlines the time frame for scheduling your appointment, and appointments close five business days prior to the examination date. They are allocated on a first-come, first-served basis.

While exact dates may vary annually, the following timeline applies to the 2025 cycle and can serve as a general planning reference.

- May 24 – Exam registration opens
- September 1 – Deadline to register for the FPGEE
- September 24 – Last day to request a new FIC or change your legal name
- October 17 – Final day to schedule or cancel your exam appointment with Pearson VUE

The NABP will issue an FPGEE Identification Card (FIC) once you have the ATT letter. This card is essential for accessing a Pearson VUE Center to take the FPGEE exam. Depending on your location, it may take up to four weeks to receive your FIC. Therefore, do not register for the exam until you confirm receipt of the FIC. Remember, there is a final deadline for scheduling, so you need to balance this risk. If your FIC is delayed, contact both the NABP and Pearson VUE immediately.

Lastly, your FPGEE score report is usually posted eight to ten weeks after the exam date. Once the score is posted and all requirements are marked complete, allow an additional four to six weeks for processing, certificate issuance, and delivery by mail. You will not get the certificate in PDF or digital form. It is only sent as a hard copy. For more details about the FPGEE exam, refer to the FPGEC Candidate Application Bulletin.

CHAPTER 4

TRANSITION: PHASE TWO

You've finished your foundational steps, verified your credentials, completed or are in the process of exams, and are nearing FPGEC certification. Now, you enter one of the most crucial and challenging phases where many international pharmacists lose momentum. This setback isn't due to a lack of qualifications but often results from poor sequencing, legal misunderstandings, or strategic misalignment.

This phase involves relocating and fulfilling US licensing requirements under the supervision of a licensed professional. The process includes managing legal systems, job markets, licensure requirements, and career planning all at once. Each decision affects your internship, residency eligibility, timeline, expenses, and visa status options.

Let's explore this phase in-depth so you know all the key points to consider when planning to move to the United States.

Section 1: What Are the Key Factors Influencing Your Move?

Before applying for an internship, selecting a state, or starting your licensure process, take a moment to consider five essential questions. These questions are crucial, strategic filters that will influence the success, efficiency, and sustainability of your transition. Each of these factors impacts your ability to navigate the US system effectively, complete necessary training, and maintain eligibility for pharmacy residency.

1. What will your legal status be upon entering the US (visa type, sponsor, work authorization)?
2. Which state(s) should you choose? Consider

internship hours and exam requirements, cost of living, licensure reciprocity, and other relevant factors.

3. Will your internship be compensated? Not all internships are paid; each state has its own labor laws and regulations.
4. Will you receive your payment directly from the residency program, or will a third party, like your university or government, sponsor you? Consider your visa type, eligibility for stipends, and whether the program provides or accepts external sponsorship. Residency stipends vary widely ($40,000–$60,000/year) for the first year of a pharmacy postgraduate residency (PGY-1) and may be higher for PGY-2.
5. What is your ultimate goal in five years?

You need to reflect carefully on these questions and provide thoughtful answers, as they will guide your next steps in this journey. Do not skip these questions; they will pave the way for your success.

Section 2: Your Legal Status in the United States

Your legal status in the United States is a crucial aspect of your transition. It determines if you can start internship hours, receive payment, qualify for residency, apply for state licensing, or remain in the country after training. Immigration status is a fundamental legal element of your career plans, not a minor detail. If you are a US citizen or permanent resident (green card holder), you can skip ahead. However, if you are an international candidate, read this section carefully. It may decide whether your training plan is feasible.

4.2.1 Work Authorization and Intern Eligibility

If you are not a permanent US resident, you need to have one of the specified statuses to work legally as a pharmacy intern or pharmacy resident in the United States:

- F-1 Student Visa (through academic programs) with optional practical training (OPT)
- H-1B Nonimmigrant Work Visa

Remember that the J-1 visa (exchange visitor visa) isn't suitable for pharmacy interns or residents. It often limits direct patient care, a key component of pharmacy practice in the US. Be cautious of programs that solely provide J-1 sponsorship unless you have verified that it permits clinical pharmacy activities.

4.2.2 The F-1 Student Visa

Most international non-US resident pharmacy graduates choose to enroll in a university-based certificate or bridging pharmacy program that provides internship training and prepares them for licensure. These programs charge tuition and do not compensate for internship hours; instead, students pay the university for supervision during their training.

- The F-1 visa will allow you to work as a pharmacy intern.
- The program offers coursework in clinical pharmacy and US practice standards.
- Internship placements / clinical rotations are at affiliated US hospitals.
- Support for FPGEE and TOEFL iBT preparation is offered.

- F-1 international students can apply for optional practical training (OPT).

When arriving in the US on an F-1 visa, it's advisable to apply for a Social Security number (SSN) within ten days. This is important because:

- You cannot get a US state ID or driver's license without an SSN.
- Pearson VUE testing centers (for NAPLEX, MPJE, or state exams) require a valid US or government-issued ID for exam entry.
- Without an SSN, you might not be added to payroll, even if you're authorized to work.

Although you can register for exams online using your NABP ID, you must present a valid US physical identification (ID) on test day to access the testing center. Plan ahead to avoid last-minute problems.

4.2.3 Optional Practical Training (OPT) – A Work Authorization

OPT is a twelve-month employment permit granted exclusively to F-1 international students to gain practical experience related to their studies in pharmacy. You should request optional practical training (OPT) authorization from your university about four to six months before graduation. This work authorization is necessary if you plan to pursue a pharmacy residency, fellowship, or any other work afterward.

Most PGY-1 pharmacy residency programs will ask applicants whether their university has filed the OPT application on their behalf. Without proof that you have applied for or already received OPT work authorization, many programs will hesitate to offer you a position because they cannot legally employ you, and most probably will not offer you an H-1B visa.

Key points about OPT:

- You should apply four to six months before graduation.
- Most PGY-1 residency programs will inquire whether your university has submitted your OPT application.
- Without OPT approval, many programs cannot legally employ you, and most will not provide H-1B sponsorship.
- Your OPT period must cover the entire duration of your PGY-1 residency, and it should be within the same state(s) where you applied for the residency program.

The processing time for optional practical training (OPT) can vary widely and sometimes takes longer than expected. This can directly affect your ability to start your PGY-1 pharmacy residency on time. Since most PGY-1 programs start at the end of June, any delay in OPT approval could threaten your start date and placement. Unlike other documents, OPT approval depends not only on your university's schedule but also on federal processing times through US Citizenship and Immigration Services (USCIS), which can change based on application volume and policy updates.

To prevent delays, it's crucial to stay well-informed and proactive. Regularly check the USCIS website for the latest updates on OPT processing times, eligibility requirements, and necessary forms. Additionally, collaborate closely with your university's international student office, as they will guide you through the internal application process, track deadlines, and provide the required recommendation (Form I-20 with OPT endorsement).

Generally, if your program ends in May or June, it's recommended to submit your OPT application by March. This provides sufficient time for review, approval, and receipt of your Employment Authorization Document (EAD). When applying for OPT, ensure that your requested authorization period covers your entire PGY-1 residency, typically from the end of June of the first year to July of the following year. Consult with your university's pharmacy program director.

Applying early for OPT is essential. A delayed OPT approval that causes you to miss your residency start could mean losing this opportunity entirely.

Start early to ensure your OPT timeline aligns with your academic graduation and residency offer.

4.2.4 H-1B Nonimmigrant Work Visa

The H-1B is a nonimmigrant, employer-sponsored visa that permits individuals who are not US citizens or permanent residents to work in specialty fields, such as pharmacy. It initially lasts up to six years, with some limited exceptions. Although the H-1B can serve as a route to long-term US employment, it is generally not accessible for training roles such as pharmacy internships and is only sometimes available for postgraduate residencies.

- If you're thinking about using an H-1B visa to fulfill your internship hours, consider the following: Most employers do not sponsor H-1B visas for internships.
- Typically, H-1B sponsorship is available only for fully licensed pharmacists in full-time roles.
- Without a US pharmacy license, your chances of obtaining H-1B sponsorship as a pharmacy intern are very low.
- Even if you satisfy all clinical and academic requirements, obtaining H-1B approval during an internship is unlikely unless you already have a license and are hired as a pharmacist, not for training.

You may need an H-1B visa for a PGY-2 residency or to continue working after OPT ends, especially if you entered the United States with an F-1 visa. H-1B sponsorship isn't guaranteed and isn't available through all pharmacy residency programs. Common issues include: a limited number of PGY-1 and PGY-2 programs that sponsor H-1B visas, employers avoiding H-1B sponsorship due to legal and cost complexities, and many programs expecting OPT approval from F-1 visa holders without offering other sponsorship options. Always check the ASHP Residency Directory or contact the residency program directly to verify their visa sponsorship policies before applying.

4.2.5 Strategic Tip

If your long-term aim is to live and work in the US, transitioning to an H-1B visa might be necessary eventually. However, avoid making it your initial plan, especially for internships or PGY-1 residencies. Instead:

- Start with an F-1 visa and OPT, which are much more accessible options.
- Apply only to residency programs that explicitly support H-1B sponsorship or accept OPT.
- Consider long-term pathways, such as employment-based green card sponsorship, if you plan to stay in the United States after completing your training.

Visa sponsorship is a significant challenge for international pharmacy graduates. Developing a practical and adaptable visa strategy is crucial for achieving your long-term goals.

Section 3: Why Your Choice of State Matters

Choosing the right state is a crucial, strategic decision for international pharmacists seeking US licensure and residency. It impacts internship requirements, licensure procedures, costs, and access to residency programs. Many candidates only consider state board of pharmacy rules, like training hours or specific exams. This can be shortsighted. The state you select affects not just your training but also your eligibility for various opportunities.

4.3.1 Questions to Consider Before Selecting a State

- Does the state offer a university with a structured internship or bridging program? If you are entering the United States on an F-1 visa, this is an essential requirement.

- Are there pharmacy residency programs within the state that actively accept or designate positions for international graduates? Some states are more receptive to foreign-trained pharmacists than others.
- Do residency programs in the state provide stipends or salaries to international applicants or accept external funding from your government or educational institution? This consideration will impact the financial viability of the opportunity.
- Does the state support licensure and training regulations that are friendly toward international candidates? Examine aspects such as internship flexibility, processing times, license portability, and long-term employment prospects.

If you choose to obtain an F-1 student visa, you will be required to relocate to the state where your university is located, and you will not be paid for the internship hours; instead, you will be paying the university. Make sure you check whether the selected state has pharmacy residency programs that either specifically offer positions to international pharmacy graduates or accept them into their sites.

4.3.2 Massachusetts as a Case Study

Massachusetts College of Pharmacy and Health Sciences (MCPHS) in Boston offers the Certificate of Advanced Pharmacy Practice Studies (CAPPS), a two-year program. This program provides a pathway to residency or licensure for pharmacists trained outside the US, but it does not guarantee a residency. The two-year course prepares students for the FPGEE exam. However, if you've already passed the exam, you can contact the university to enroll in a shorter, one-year program instead, which can help lower tuition costs. You can reach out to the university even if the program is not currently listed on their website.

The state of Massachusetts has several residency programs that offer designated positions for international applicants. For example, Brigham and Women's Hospital in Boston, St. Elizabeth's Medical Center, and Tufts Medicine MelroseWakefield Hospital in Melrose each have PGY-1 and PGY-2 residency tracks specifically allocated for international pharmacy graduates. These programs are listed in the ASHP Residency Directory - the American Society of Health-System Pharmacists' database of accredited residency programs.

Although Massachusetts hosts several pharmacy residency programs for international pharmacists and offers a pharmacy bridging certificate program, these residencies do not accept applications from international pharmacists and do not provide stipends or H-1B visa sponsorship unless a university or government agency sponsors the applicant.

4.3.3 Other University-Based Programs

Several universities outside Massachusetts provide bridging certificate programs tailored for international pharmacy graduates. These programs can be a pathway to complete internship hours, acquire US clinical experience, and potentially qualify for a PGY-1 residency. Examples include:

- University of Southern California (USC) – Graduate Certificate in Advanced Pharmacy Practice
    - While this program provides advanced clinical

pharmacy training, from my experience, there is currently no information available regarding the residency placement success of international students in California

- University of Arizona – Certificate in Advanced Clinical Pharmacy Practice
    - This program may have a structure similar to MCPHS, possibly including clinical rotations and preparation for the FPGEE. However, residency placements and stipends should be confirmed directly with the university, as access for international students may vary by year and sponsorship.
- UC San Diego Health Science International – Bridge to Residency Pharmacy Program
    - A similar case to USC.

For more information about residency programs that have designated positions for international applicants, refer to the reference section.

4.3.4 Obtain Pharmacy Intern Licensure

After entering the US and verifying your work authorization (such as F-1/OPT, H-1B, or green card), the next important step is to apply for a pharmacy intern license in your chosen state. This license allows you to work under the supervision of a pharmacist and begin accumulating the required internship hours for that state.

NABP does not have a centralized intern license application. Each state Board of Pharmacy (BOP) maintains its own application form, document requirements, submission procedures, and fees. You must submit your application directly to the board in the state where you intend to practice.

Most state boards require at the least: proof of FPGEC certification or progress (like completed TOEFL and ECE, and submitted NABP application), a Social Security number (SSN), a US address (temporary addresses may be accepted in some states), a criminal background check or fingerprinting, submission of official documents such as transcripts, passport, and degree or license attestations (usually in sealed envelopes), and application fees ranging from $50 to $250, depending on the state.

Processing intern licenses can take four to twelve weeks, depending on the state. It's best to apply early, ideally after receiving your FPGEC certificate and securing legal US work status. If you're participating in a university-based bridging program, ask the school's administration to assist with the license application, as they usually have experience with the state's licensing procedures.

Lastly, confirm the internship hour tracking policy with the BOP and the university program director, and document all communications.

4.3.5 Selecting Your Internship Clinical Rotations

Should you opt to enroll in a pharmacy bridging certificate program, your clinical rotations will significantly influence your residency application. In addition to satisfying internship prerequisites, these rotations serve as a direct indication of your clinical preparedness and may either enhance or diminish your competitiveness within the residency selection process.

Choose high-impact clinical settings whenever possible, selecting rotations at high-acuity hospitals, such as Level III Trauma Centers, academic medical centers, or major teaching hospitals.

These settings provide:

- Exposure to more complex patient cases.
- Opportunities for interprofessional collaboration.
- Institutional protocols that meet residency standards.
- Recommendation letters from your preceptor rotations for the future residency.

Avoid filling your internship rotations with community or general inpatient pharmacy experiences, as these are not required for international pharmacy graduates and are mainly part of the PharmD program. These experiences are considered basic and won't set your application apart.

Furthermore, it is essential to diligently consider the range of rotation types provided by the university and to prioritize specialized rotations such as intensive care, cardiology, thrombosis, infectious disease, pediatrics, oncology, or whichever area aligns most closely with your interests.

To ensure your experience meets PGY-1 expectations, review the rotation categories mandated by PGY-1 programs, typically encompassing eight core areas. If feasible, complete some of these rotations during your internship to demonstrate alignment with requirements and preparedness.

Many programs allow students to request specific rotation sites and specialties. If your preferred options are not immediately available, you can often delay your program start date so that faculty can review and accommodate your request. Targeting these advanced experiences can strengthen your profile and improve your chances of securing a residency position.

4.3.6 Completing Your Licensure Exam

Once you've finished your internship hours, the next essential step is to pass two licensure exams: the North American Pharmacist Licensure Examination (NAPLEX) and one of the following law exams, either the Multistate Pharmacy Jurisprudence Examination (MPJE) or a state-specific law exam like the CPJE in California or Virginia's Pharmacy Law Exam. You can purchase both exams from the NABP website.

4.3.7 Other Practical Factors to Consider

While your primary focus may be on residency opportunities and licensure pathways, there are several practical and logistical factors that should also influence your decision when selecting a state. These considerations do not directly relate to securing a residency, but they can significantly impact your training experience, financial circumstances, and long-term objectives.

- Almost every state requires you to complete internship training hours before you can sit for the NAPLEX and the MPJE, the CPJE (California), the Virginia Pharmacy Law Exam, or the Arkansas Jurisprudence Exam. Most states mandate between 1,500 and 2,080 hours.
- A few states allow partial credit for foreign work experience; for example, California does not, while New York and Texas may grant partial credit after evaluation. If you are planning for residency, then I would not recommend transferring these work experience credits. Certain states

require that all internship hours be earned in the US under a licensed pharmacist preceptor.

- California is the only state that does not accept NABP's license transfer program. If you plan to practice there, you may need to take the NAPLEX again. Be sure to review the California Board of Pharmacy's requirements in detail before committing.
- Each state board of pharmacy, not NABP, determines:
  - The number of hours you must complete.
  - How those hours must be documented.
  - Whether any hours earned abroad will be accepted.
  - Whether you must be registered as an intern before you begin accumulating hours.
- Other factors to consider:
  - The cost of living in the state and city where you will train or study.
  - Availability of affordable housing and transportation options.
  - State income tax obligations, which can significantly affect your net income.
  - The overall job market and demand for pharmacists after you complete your training (refer to the reference section).
  - Opportunities for sponsorship through H-1B or employment-based green cards (if relevant).
  - Proximity to professional networks, cultural

communities, or support systems that are important to you.

Section 4: What Is Your Ultimate Goal?

Before making any decisions about licensure or training, it's crucial to define your long-term goal. This clarity will shape every strategic choice—from the state you choose to move to, the visa you select, and the programs you decide to pursue. Ask yourself: Am I aiming to finish my training and go back to my home country, or do I want to establish a long-term pharmacy career in the United States?

If your goal is to return home after completing a postgraduate residency, you will probably conclude your training after PGY-1 or PGY-2. Focus on gaining high-quality US clinical experience, securing strong references, and developing skills that match the healthcare system in your home country. Prioritize rotations and experiences that mirror the practice environments you intend to work in upon return.

Conversely, if you plan to stay in the US, start preparing early—ideally from the moment you consider which state to move to and which pathway to follow. Long-term retention in the US requires more than just clinical qualifications. It involves strategic immigration planning, career development, and establishing early relationships with potential employers. Start planning now in these key areas:

- **Visa Strategy:** Explore options beyond OPT, such as transitioning to an H-1B visa or pursuing employment-based green cards. Keep in mind that not all employers can sponsor visas; your eligibility may depend on your training location, the institutions you partner with, and current visa policies.

- **Residency Site Advantage:** Some residents receive permanent positions at their PGY-1 or PGY-2 training sites. Be proactive by expressing interest early and cultivating strong relationships with preceptors, mentors, and department leaders.
- **Professional Networking:** Start building your network from your first rotation. Use mentors, career fairs, alumni groups, and professional conferences intentionally. The ASHP Midyear Clinical Meeting is the largest US event for making professional connections and meeting potential employers.
- **Job Market Readiness:** Target training in high-demand specialties. Stay updated on job trends, salary expectations, and licensing portability across states. Begin preparing your resume, developing your portfolio, and applying for jobs early in your PGY-2 year. In addition, attend national conferences like the ASHP Midyear to participate in the residency showcase, meet program directors, and connect with employers at the career fair.

If you prefer to continue training and your interest lies in research, academia, or the pharmaceutical industry, you may also consider pursuing:

- Fellowships in clinical pharmacology, health outcomes, or industry leadership.

- Postdoctoral training in academic or clinical specialties.

These opportunities may offer specialized credentials, leadership development, or access to career trajectories that are not typically accessible through conventional residency programs.

Whether you're aiming to return home after residency or build a lasting pharmacy career in the US, defining your goal early keeps your journey focused and efficient.

Your objective shapes your path and dictates every decision, whether it's licensing, location, or visa. Regularly revisit your plan, as expanding clinical experience and new opportunities can shift your goals. Stay adaptable yet purposeful. Achieving long-term success starts with clear, long-term vision.

Lastly, keep in mind that planning is especially critical if you are on an H-1B visa, since you are only permitted to remain in the US for thirty to sixty days after your last day of employment. Always refer to USCIS for the most up-to-date information on visa regulations and timelines (see appendix D).

CHAPTER 5

ADVANCEMENT: PHASE THREE

As we transition from phase two to phase three, it's important to emphasize the critical role of passing your pharmacy licensure exams not only as a licensing requirement but also as a strategic move that impacts your residency success and career growth. Whenever possible, complete both licensure exams before starting your PGY-1 residency. This decision can significantly reduce stress, enhance your clinical performance, and allow you to enter residency with full professional credentials.

It is worth mentioning that many pharmacy graduates in the US and internationally take the NAPLEX and MPJE (or other state law exam) during the first ninety days of residency, but doing so under pressure can be risky. Here's why preparing early is smarter:

- The initial weeks of PGY-1 are intense, with onboarding, patient care, shift coverage, presentations, and ongoing evaluations, all while adjusting to a new clinical setting.
- Studying for licensure exams at this time splits your focus and can hurt both your test results and clinical learning.
- Being fully licensed before residency offers more independence, earns trust from preceptors, and allows you to contribute more effectively from the start.

If passing both exams before residency isn't feasible, prioritize completing the NAPLEX first, as it may limit clinical flexibility while you study for the MPJE or state law exam. However, please note that the verification process (degree, FPGEC certificate, and internship hours) for eligibility to sit for the exam varies by state and may take several weeks or longer to complete. Refer to the NABP website and BOP in your selected state.

Section 1: Pharmacy Residency Application Process

To start the pharmacy residency application process, familiarize yourself with two key platforms: PhORCAS— the Pharmacy Online Residency Centralized Application Service—and the Match, formerly called the ASHP Resident Matching Program, managed by National Matching Services Inc. PhORCAS is a web-based system that simplifies and standardizes applications by allowing you to submit your personal statement, recommendation letters, transcripts, and CV all in one secure place. It also streamlines communication between applicants and programs, ensuring consistent receipt and evaluation of applications. The Match handles the placement of residency positions for PGY-1 and PGY-2 programs, providing a fair and transparent process that helps candidates secure preferred positions while assisting programs in filling openings with suitable candidates. This matching system is similar to those used in other health fields like medicine, dentistry, optometry, psychology, and podiatry, and is regarded as the standard for fairness and efficiency.

The ASHP oversees the rules of the Match, maintaining consistency and integrity across institutions, while National Matching Services Inc. manages daily operations such as rank processing, algorithms, and notifications on behalf of the ASHP. Understanding how these systems work together is essential for building a successful residency application plan.

5.1.1 Starting Your Pharmacy Residency Application

The residency application process is often thought to start with creating a PhORCAS account and submitting your documents, but in reality, you should begin much earlier. Start preparing for residency while you're still an intern. Early preparation provides a key advantage by allowing more time to gain clinical experience, secure strong recommendations (US-based preceptors), and develop your personal narrative. Crucially, it also gives you the opportunity to explore residency programs without the pressure of looming deadlines.

One of the best ways to start early is by attending the ASHP Midyear Clinical Meeting, even if you're not yet applying. This event features the ASHP Residency Showcase, the largest pharmacy residency exhibit worldwide, bringing together residency programs, preceptors, current residents, and future applicants in a single, impactful setting. Attending offers direct insight into what programs expect from candidates, how they differ in culture, focus, and structure, and which programs best match your clinical interests and long-term goals. Engaging with programs early helps you make informed decisions, avoid mismatched applications, and position yourself strategically for the PhORCAS submission.

Attending the student and resident poster presentations during Midyear is equally vital. These sessions showcase various research projects, clinical innovations, and practice models that different residency programs emphasize. You will discover:

- The key topics highlighted in different programs.
- How residents utilize clinical skills in practical settings.
- Which institutions match your interests or future aspirations.

Attending both the ASHP Residency Showcase and poster presentations not only offers early insight into the residency landscape but also helps you understand each program's academic focus, research environment, and clinical identity before you become an applicant. Attending Midyear as a student intern shows proactive planning. It influences your decisions, fuels your clinical interests, and allows you to craft more tailored, informed applications when the time comes.

Researching past residency programs is another crucial, strategic step. It's essential to determine which programs are open to hiring non-US citizens and are willing to sponsor H-1B work authorization or accept your OPT.

Before applying, review the previous year's participating programs in the official ASHP Match Program directory. This directory helps you understand the types and locations of available programs, filter based on training focus or institution location, and identify programs that may accept F-1/OPT candidates or sponsor H-1B visas.

Keep in mind, not all programs sponsor H-1B visas or accept OPT employment. Be sure to research thoroughly or contact programs directly to verify their visa policies. Residency is competitive but strategic. Targeting programs based on clinical fit and immigration feasibility is often overlooked but essential. Being proactive can save you time, money, and missed opportunities.

If you have completed this part of researching residency programs with international tracks before moving to the US, well done. You have followed the guidance from chapter four, section three. Therefore, your search is now more focused.

Finally, remember to utilize the support resources offered by your university. If you're enrolled in a US-based bridging or certificate program, contact your program director or international office early on. They usually have knowledge about residency programs that have previously accepted international graduates and might have direct contacts with sites willing to sponsor OPT or H-1B visas. Although they cannot guarantee placements, their advice can save you time by steering you away from unsuitable programs. Make sure to take advantage of every resource at your disposal, especially those connected to your current academic environment.

5.1.2 The PhORCAS Timeline

This section assumes you've already researched suitable residency programs that match your clinical interests and, importantly, support your legal stay and work authorization in the US, whether through F-1 OPT or H-1B visa sponsorship. Without this, even a strong application might be rejected for reasons beyond the applicant's control.

Understanding the residency application timeline is crucial, especially for international graduates who often underestimate the importance of early preparation. The Pharmacy Online Residency Centralized Application Service (PhORCAS) opens at the beginning of November each year. When the PhORCAS portal opens, successful candidates who have planned ahead are ready to submit their applications, while others are just starting to explore the programs and their requirements to begin the application process.

If you're currently doing a pharmacy internship at a US hospital or clinical site, you might be working alongside PharmD students from US pharmacy schools. These students are usually in their fourth year (P4) and apply for residency through PhORCAS in November, even though they graduate in May. Many of them are still completing their first or second rotations when they start applying.

These applicants:

- Submit their applications before graduation and interview while they are still students, and they can match before getting their license or finishing their rotations.
- Don't wait until May to graduate before applying because that would delay their start until July the next year, wasting a whole year. As an international graduate, you face the same timeline. To stay competitive, plan early, prepare in advance, and be ready to apply in November, regardless of your current licensing or internship status.
- Take the NAPLEX/MPJE during their first ninety days of residency.

The PhORCAS application cycle begins in early November and usually runs until December 31. This is the primary period for submitting applications for PGY-1 residency programs. However, remember that each program sets its own deadline; some may close earlier, while others may extend into early January. Always verify deadlines in PhORCAS and the ASHP Residency Directory as late submissions are not accepted.

In addition to preparing your PhORCAS application, you must register for the Match through the National Matching Services (NMS) system, which is mandatory. Programs will only review candidates who are officially registered. After registering, you will receive a match code number that must be entered into your PhORCAS profile.

After you have submitted your applications, most programs send interview invitations in January and February. Interviews are mostly virtual, but some sites may offer in-person visits. Following interviews, you need to submit your rank order list through the Match system, listing only the residency sites where you were interviewed. Programs do the same. Both sides submit their rankings independently, and the Match algorithm pairs applicants and programs based on mutual preferences.

You will enter Phase I of the Match, with results usually announced in mid-March. If you do not match in Phase I, you can participate in Phase II, which provides a second chance to apply for unfilled positions through a shorter and faster process.

Make sure you don't miss the PhORCAS cycle. Be fully prepared to submit your application when the system opens in November, even if your internship has just started. This is common practice for US graduates, and as an international applicant, following the same schedule is essential to stay competitive. But timing alone isn't enough. You must also complete your internship hours and get them verified by your state board at least a couple of months before residency begins. Most residencies start in late June or early July, and many will require proof that your licensure process is progressing. Delays in hours can lead to licensing delays and possibly the withdrawal of your offer.

The timeline below outlines when and how to meet deadlines confidently and avoid last-minute errors.

Important considerations for international pharmacy graduates before applying to PhORCAS:

- Ensure you review the start and end dates of your US internship or bridging certificate program.
- Then, align those dates with the fixed US residency calendar. PhORCAS opens in early November, and most residencies start in late June or early July.
- To stay on schedule, complete and verify your internship hours at least one to two months before residency begins. This buffer period allows for:
    - State board verification, NAPLEX, and MPJE exams;
    - Licensure processing;
    - Visa or OPT paperwork if needed; and
    - Relocation or onboarding arrangements.

Many candidates forget to do this, risking program withdrawal if they're not licensed or prepared by July. Plan your application timeline around your program schedule, never the reverse.

Preparing for the PhORCAS required documents:

August

- Start preparing your CV and personal statement.
- Contact your clinical site preceptors to request recommendation letters for your residency, ensuring they agree to provide them. You will need three recommendation letters.
- Review the ASHP Residency Directory to research

programs and be familiar with their previous requirements, such as assays or presentations.

- Participate in any available residency preparation workshops; some sites offer virtual sessions for PharmD students. These invitations are often received through earlier communication with the residency program director or via their university or through the residency program website, so stay informed about these opportunities (throughout the year).

September

- Finalize application materials.
- Confirm references and gather transcripts (you may need to upload your FPGEC certificate).
- Customize personal statements for each program.
- Prepare for submission once the portal opens.

Early November (PhORCAS opens)

- Review the ASHP Residency Directory to confirm whether the program you're interested in participates in the Match.
- Check the program requirements for any updates from last year.
- Monitor each program's specific deadline, as some may close before December 31.
- Submit your applications early to ensure timely submission.

December

- These are the final weeks to submit applications.
- Most program deadlines are between Dec 15–31.

January – February (Phase I)

- Interview invitations are sent out.
- Prepare for virtual or optional in-person interviews.
- Begin developing a ranking strategy.

February - March

- Submit your rank order list (only for programs that interviewed you).
- Programs submit theirs.
- Match Day (Phase I): usually mid-March.
- If unmatched, enter Phase II for the remaining positions.

5.1.3 Developing a Competitive PhORCAS Profile

We've already covered many of these elements, but now let's unify them in one place. This section serves as your checklist and reference for developing a competitive PhORCAS application that showcases not just your qualifications but also your strategy, preparation, and intentions.

By this point, I assume your CV is already distinctive because it highlights something most US applicants cannot claim. You made the bold choice to leave your home country, step out of your comfort zone, and pursue one of the most challenging careers in the US. That alone speaks volumes about your mindset.

However, a strong CV is only part of the broader story. What we've constructed together throughout this roadmap is much deeper—and now it's time to demonstrate it.

Let's review the key strategic pillars that distinguish you:

1. You Selected the Appropriate States

   Your application wasn't random; you chose states that align with your licensure timeline and enable you to complete internship hours legally and efficiently.

2. You Focused on the Right Programs

   You evaluated programs based on clinical relevance and immigration policies—favoring those that accept F-1 OPT or sponsor H-1B visas. This was a deliberate choice, not guesswork. Keep in mind that your OPT should cover the duration of your residency,

3. You Coordinated Your Internship Rotations with PGY-1 Requirements

   Instead of selecting rotations arbitrarily, you tailored your internship to include core areas mandated by PGY-1 programs, such as internal medicine, critical care, infectious diseases, or ambulatory care, aligning your training with your targeted residencies. You can find the required rotations listed on the website in the pharmacy residency PGY-1 manual.

4. You Secured US Preceptors

Through your academic or clinical internship placements, you have US preceptors who know your skills, have observed your clinical work, and can write effective recommendation letters. Their support is more influential than transcripts.

5. You Completed Your Licensure Exams

   You've either already passed or are strategically preparing to take the NAPLEX and MPJE before residency starts (see appendix E).

Section 2: Pharmacy Residency Programs (PGY-1 and PGY-2)

This section examines historical trends in pharmacy residency programs that have accepted international pharmacy graduates and explains why some sites are more likely to sponsor visas than others. In addition, it will provide you with key insights into the structure of residency programs, such as how to interpret program descriptions, what staffing and scheduling models to watch, and why some rotation titles might be ambiguous. These practical details are often overlooked but can significantly affect your experience, workload, and chances of completing the program successfully while managing licensure and immigration timelines.

Programs affiliated with major universities generally have higher acceptance rates for international candidates because they often possess an established international office dedicated to managing visa sponsorship and processing H-1B applications. This administrative support makes a significant difference.

Without an international office, most hospital-based or community programs typically lack the internal capacity or legal resources to file a visa petition like an H-1B or handle OPT employment processes. Consequently, they are much less likely to admit international graduates, regardless of the strength of their application.

In summary, residency programs without the necessary visa support infrastructure are unlikely to accept international applicants.

Based on historical match data, discussions with program directors, and publicly available information, the following US states have a history of pharmacy residency programs that have accepted international pharmacy graduates: Illinois, Florida, New York, Massachusetts, North Carolina, Arizona, Oregon, Pennsylvania, Utah, Washington, Texas, South Carolina, Pennsylvania, and Virginia. These states feature either university programs experienced in sponsoring H-1B visas or PharmD-granting institutions that admit international candidates into bridging programs, which can lead to placement in affiliated PGY-1 sites. Refer to chapter three regarding the state of Massachusetts.

While not every program in these states is international-friendly, your likelihood of success is considerably higher in these states compared to states with limited academic infrastructure or predominantly community-based residency sites.

From my firsthand experience and verification in past application cycles, these residency programs have either accepted or demonstrated openness to accepting international pharmacy graduates:

- Memorial Hospital West – Pembroke Pines, FL
- University of Illinois Chicago, Retzky College of Pharmacy – Chicago, IL
- Brigham and Women's Hospital – Boston, MA
- Boston Medical Center (formerly St. Elizabeth's Medical Center) – Brighton, MA
- Tufts Medicine MelroseWakefield Hospital – Medford, MA
- Houston Methodist Hospital – Houston, TX
- Providence ElderPlace – Portland, OR
- New York-Presbyterian Brooklyn Methodist Hospital – Brooklyn, NY
- Intermountain Medical Center – Murray, UT
- Duquesne University School of Pharmacy – Pittsburgh, PA
- University of Arizona College of Pharmacy-affiliated residency programs – Tucson, AZ
- University of Washington Medical Center – Seattle, WA
    - *(Note: Only if your OPT is issued in Washington)
- Massachusetts General Hospital – Boston, MA
    - *(Note: Only if your OPT is issued in Massachusetts)
- Virginia Commonwealth University – Richmond, VA
    - *(Note: Only if your OPT is issued in Virginia)

- Medical University of South Carolina (MUSC) – Charleston, SC
    - *(Note: Only if your OPT is issued in South Carolina)

Some programs only consider international graduates if their OPT was issued within the same state as the residency site. Additionally, while a program may accept you for PGY-1, they are not obligated to offer you a PGY-2 position—even if you express a strong interest in staying. Many institutions that accept international graduates for PGY-1 do not provide visa support or extend employment beyond the first year, especially if H-1B sponsorship is not part of their policy. Always verify eligibility and visa policy with the residency program coordinator before applying. Don't assume you will progress from PGY-1 to PGY-2. Confirm it directly.

In California, the prospects for international pharmacy graduates are particularly unclear. While the state hosts two major institutions offering bridging programs—University of Southern California (USC) and UC San Diego Health Sciences—there is no documented evidence of international graduates being accepted into California PGY-1 residency programs with visa sponsorship. Despite the educational infrastructure, we have not found cases where California programs have successfully sponsored foreign graduates for OPT or H-1B visas during residency. If you're thinking about California, proceed carefully.

In addition to the visa uncertainties, California requires its own pharmacy law exam (CPJE) instead of the MPJE. If you get licensed in California and later move to another state, you will probably need to take that state's law exam. Additionally,

California does not participate in the NABP license transfer (reciprocity) process.

Be aware that California could restrict your mobility and residency options as an international graduate.

5.2.1 Understanding Residency Program Structure

Every accredited residency program has a program manual—a formal document that details rotation structure, learning objectives, staffing roles, and evaluation standards. While it's not always publicly available, you can request it during interviews or prior to signing a commitment letter. Review it carefully and ask questions such as: How are rotations organized? How is staffing determined? How many weekends are required per month? Are overnight or on-call duties expected? Is licensure needed before staffing begins? These factors are important, especially when managing licensure timelines, visa hours, and adjusting to US clinical culture, which may differ from your previous experiences.

For international graduates, adjustment involves more than clinical skills; it includes cultural and regulatory differences. You should anticipate longer shifts, varying expectations from preceptors, and strict documentation standards. Protocols must be adhered to exactly, with a culture that values independent decision-making, quick critical thinking, and collaboration across disciplines. You might also face different norms regarding punctuality, time management, email communication, and assertiveness in clinical settings, each influencing how your performance is viewed. Recognizing these hidden expectations early helps you select programs that align with your clinical objectives and ease your integration into the US healthcare system. The program manual isn't just bureaucratic paperwork; it offers a glimpse into your daily routine.

Sometimes, clinical rotation titles can be unclear or misleading. For example, in PGY-1 program schedules, the term "Advanced Clinical Pharmacy Practice" often appears. Initially, it might seem to be a senior-level clinical rotation emphasizing advanced therapeutic decision-making. However, many international applicants find that this block is mainly operational, involving staffing in nonclinical or transitional areas such as inpatient central pharmacy, clean room compounding, medication dispensing, and sterile product preparation.

Although these are valuable learning areas, they are mainly operational, not focused on clinical intervention. If your primary goal is to gain strong clinical experience, or if you are already familiar with an operational background, this rotation may offer limited benefits. It's essential to inquire about the program's definition of "advanced practice" and whether clinical decision-making is a key component of the role or if it primarily focuses on service-oriented tasks.

Staffing is essential in most PGY-1 residency programs, but how often you're scheduled varies widely. The three main models are: every other weekend, every third weekend, or once a month. Some programs have alternating blocks, such as one month without staffing, then one with weekend shifts. Others may require both weekend and evening coverage, especially in community or inpatient settings.

International residents often underestimate the physical and emotional exhaustion from weekend staffing, particularly when preparing for licensure exams or adapting to a new healthcare system. When staffing occurs every other weekend, it can disrupt study schedules, attending required conferences such as ASHP, or licensure exams like the NAPLEX or MPJE.

Ask the residency program coordinator:

- What is the weekend staffing model?
- Are weekend duties solely operational, or do they include clinical services?
- Will I be expected to staff before earning full pharmacist licensure?

Residency structure isn't just about learning; it also involves workload, sustainability, and how well it aligns with your licensure timeline. Don't consider only the hospital's reputation; also pay attention to the responsibilities you'll have during each rotation. The program manual details all of this. Think of it as the essential document you must review before making a commitment. It typically includes rotation schedules, staffing models, weekend expectations, on-call services, licensure deadlines, and evaluation criteria. Often, you can find this manual or a sample on the program's website. If it's not available, ask for it before or during the interview. Read it carefully and compare it with other programs. Evaluate whether the workload, structure, and expectations are manageable for you, especially given visa requirements, licensure deadlines, and cultural adjustments. A program may appear impressive, but your success depends on whether it's truly structured to support your specific needs.

5.2.2 Final Considerations on Residency Salary, Sponsorship, and Overtime: What You Need to Know Before Choosing a Program

As you narrow your residency program choices, consider not only clinical fit and visa requirements but also the financial and logistical aspects of each option. This is particularly crucial for international pharmacy graduates, whether you're sponsored or on OPT.

As previously noted, if your residency is sponsored by your government, your salary will be paid by that sponsor rather than by the hospital or program. In such cases, your financial arrangements, including housing, stipends, and benefits, are determined by your sponsorship agreement. Conversely, if you're not sponsored and are working under F-1 OPT, your salary comes directly from the residency program, making it essential to thoroughly understand your employment contract.

From my experience, international pharmacists on OPT often overlook important questions such as:

- Are you eligible for overtime pay?
- If not paid for overtime, will you receive compensatory time off?
- Are conferences (like ASHP Midyear) considered part of paid work or attended on your own time?
- Who pays for your health insurance?

Most sponsored international residents I've seen are not compensated for overtime or time spent at mandatory conferences.

These activities are viewed as part of your government-funded training, not paid labor.

Before signing any offer letter, clarify your employment expectations. Whether you're on OPT or self-funded, every paid or unpaid hour has financial and legal implications.

CHAPTER 6

MATCH RATES, TRENDS, AND STRATEGIC INSIGHT

Before exploring residency match trends, let's first examine key data on the overall pharmacy workforce in the United States. Although this information isn't specific to residency applicants, it provides valuable context—particularly for internationally graduated pharmacists—by highlighting the number of practicing pharmacists in the US who obtained their degrees abroad.

Based on the October 2022 NABP E-Profile Aggregate Data for the Pharmacy Workforce Center, there were over 337,000 pharmacists with active profiles in the US. Of these, 319,914 obtained their pharmacy degree from a US institution, 12,971 from a non-US pharmacy school, and 4,117 had no recorded degree location. This indicates that roughly 3.8 percent of the US pharmacy workforce consists of foreign-educated pharmacists.

It's important to note that this statistic covers all licensed pharmacists, not solely those applying for residency. It includes:

- US citizens or permanent residents who studied abroad;
- Foreign-trained pharmacists who completed licensure without a residency;
- Individuals in retail, regulatory, industry, or nonclinical roles; and
- Candidates who may not be dependent on OPT or H-1B sponsorship.

This figure does not show the number of international graduates applying for PGY-1 residency programs. Instead, it indicates that the actual number of foreign-trained pharmacists entering the PGY-1 Match on F-1 or H-1B visas is much lower and mostly not documented in public records.

Section 1: The 2025 ASHP Resident Matching Statistics

The 2025 ASHP Resident Matching Program, covering both Phase I and Phase II, offers a valuable overview of current residency trends (Table 1).

Table (1) 2025 ASHP Resident Match Statistics - Phase I and II Combined					
Level	**Program**	***Positions Offered**	**Positions Filled**	**Positions Unfilled**	**Fill Rate (%)**
PGY-1	1,707	4,259	4,063	164	95.1
PGY-2	1,310	1,703	1,496	181	87.8
Total	3,017	5,962	5,559	345	93.2

**The Positions Offered in the ASHP Match reports might not match the sum of "Positions Filled" and "Positions Unfilled." This is because some programs withdraw, students commit early, and the Match process has its own reporting definitions.*

In 2025, there were 5,962 residency positions available across the US, with 345 remaining unfilled after both application phases. These unfilled roles often present opportunities, especially in less competitive specialties or underserved regions.

At first glance, the 2025 Match results appear promising, with 5,962 positions offered and fill rates exceeding 95 percent for PGY-1 and 87.8 percent for PGY-2. However, for international graduates, the reality is much narrower—and numbers alone don't fully capture the situation.

For the 2025 cycle, only six PGY-1 positions nationwide and six PGY-2 positions at a single institution were set aside for international applicants. These spots, usually filled by non-U.S. citizens with a U.S. PharmD degree and often sponsored by their home countries, account for just 0.14% of the 4,259 PGY-1 positions available and 0.35% of the 1,703 PGY-2 positions.

In total, only about 0.2% (12 out of 5,962) of all residency positions were opened to international applicants, a stark contrast to the thousands of positions shown in the match statistics.

For international graduates, especially those on F-1 OPT or requiring H-1B sponsorship, this drastically changes the landscape: the residency match may appear numerically large, but realistic access is severely restricted.

Furthermore, if we look into more detailed statistics published by the Match, the actual number of international pharmacy graduates who applied and successfully matched was very small. In the PGY-1 cycle, only eighteen applicants were from Lebanese American University (LAU), and thirty-three were from other foreign, non-ACPE-accredited pharmacy schools. Of these, just six LAU applicants and seven foreign-trained applicants matched into PGY-1 residency programs, resulting in match rates of 50 percent and 26.9 percent, respectively (Table 2).

It is important to note that the Lebanese American University (LAU) is categorized separately in the Match statistics due to its unique status as the sole pharmacy institution outside the United States holding full ACPE accreditation. Although other international universities may possess ACPE certification, such certification does not possess the same evaluative significance as full ACPE accreditation in the context of program equivalency or residency competitiveness.

Table (2) 2025 ASHP Matching Statistics for International Pharmacy Graduates - Phase I and II Combined							
Application Group	Registered	Early commit	Active with list	Matched	Unmatched	Match Rate - active list (%)	*Match Rate - registered (%)
PGY-1							
LAU	18	-	12	6	6	50	33.3
Foreign Schools	33	-	26	7	19	26.9	21.2
PGY-2							
LAU	3	1	2	1	1	50	67
Foreign Schools	1	0	1	1	0	100	100

**Match Rate (%) for registered candidates, including those accepted through early commitment*

During the PGY-2 cycle, only three LAU applicants participated, with one matching and one early commit, and just one foreign-trained applicant from a non-ACPE school registered and matched. However, it's important to clarify that these figures refer to international graduates, not necessarily non-US citizens (Table 2).

Many applicants from non-US pharmacy schools may be US citizens or permanent residents, including those who returned to the US after studying abroad. Therefore, the actual number of international graduates applying for residencies while on F-1 visas or seeking H-1B sponsorship remains unknown but is certainly smaller than these limited figures.

Section 2: The 2021 – 2024 ASHP Resident Matching Statistics

Between 2021 and 2024, PGY-1 residency positions in the US consistently achieved high fill rates, ranging from 95.6 percent to 99.3 percent, despite an increase in available spots. Conversely, PGY-2 programs continued to face lower fill rates, fluctuating between 88.9 percent and 97.3 percent, indicating growing saturation and selectivity at this advanced stage (Table 3).

Table (3) Overview of ASHP Resident Match Statistics 2021-2024: Phases I & II Combined

Year	Level	Program	Positions Offered	Positions Filled	Positions Unfilled	Fill Rate (%)
2021	PGY-1	1,578	4,042	4,015	19	99.3
	PGY-2	1,131	1,492	1,452	34	97.3
	Total	2,709	5,534	5,467	53	98.8
2022	PGY-1	1,633	4,242	4,152	74	97.9
	PGY-2	1,197	1,585	1,409	146	88.9
	Total	2,830	5,827	5,561	220	95.4
2023	PGY-1	1,672	4,249	4,099	114	96.5
	PGY-2	1,214	1,608	1,438	142	89.4
	Total	2,886	5,857	5,537	256	94.5

2024	PGY-1	1,694	4,270	4,081	150	95.6
	PGY-2	1,227	1,626	1,490	119	91.6
	Total	2,921	5,896	5,571	269	94.5

A detailed look at international pharmacy graduates, particularly from the Lebanese American University (LAU) and other non-ACPE-accredited foreign schools, reveals a stark disparity (Tables 4 and 5).

PGY-1 applicants from LAU experienced fluctuating match rates, peaking at 85.7 percent in 2023 but dropping to 50 percent in 2024. Those from foreign schools had consistently low match rates, between 15.6 percent and 42.9 percent over four years (Table 5).

Table (4) Overview of 2021–2024 International Pharmacy Graduates' Match Statistics (LAU) — Phases I & II Combined

Year	Registered	Early commit	Active with list	Matched	Unmatched	Match Rate - active list (%)	*Match Rate - registered (%)
PGY-1							
2024	11	-	10	5	5	50	45.5
2023	9	-	7	6	1	85.7	66.7
2022	12	-	11	8	3	72.7	66.7
2021	20	-	17	6	11	35.3	30

PGY-2							
2024	6	1	4	2	2	50	50
2023	5	2	3	0	3	0	40
2022	4	1	3	2	1	66.7	75
2021	1	0	0	0	0	0	0

**Match Rate (%) for registered candidates, including those accepted through early commitment*

For PGY-2 international graduates, while initial data might seem promising, such as a 100 percent match rate in 2023 for foreign schools, these figures are based on very small sample sizes, often just one or two applicants (Table 5). This makes the data statistically insignificant and not indicative of broader trends. A single success or failure can greatly alter the percentage, limiting its predictive value.

These figures underscore an ongoing reality: Securing a US residency for international graduates remains highly competitive, with little room for error. Applicants should approach this goal with a realistic view of their chances, especially during PGY-2 cycles, and focus on detailed planning, visa strategies, program eligibility, and understanding historical match patterns for international graduates.

Table (5) Overview of 2021–2024 International Pharmacy Graduates' Match Statistics (Foreign Pharmacy School) — Phases I & II Combined							
Year	**Registered**	**Early commit**	**Active with list**	**Matched**	**Unmatched**	**Match Rate - active list (%)**	***Match Rate - registered (%)**
PGY-1							
2024	21	-	14	4	10	28.6	19
2023	29	-	21	9	12	42.9	31
2022	35	-	24	7	17	29.2	20
2021	55	-	32	5	27	15.6	9.1
PGY-2							
2024	5	0	4	3	1	75	60
2023	1	0	1	1	0	100	100
2022	2	0	2	1	1	50	50
2021	8	0	8	5	3	62.5	62.5

**Match Rate (%) for registered candidates, including those accepted through early commitment*

Overall, residency programs are competitive for all applicants, but international candidates with temporary visas face stiffer competition and a narrower window. Nevertheless, matching is still achievable. Success largely depends on approaching the process with a strategic, precise, and realistic understanding of eligibility.

How to Navigate This Reality

- Consider each potential program as a unique research project. Check their visa policies, OPT/H-1B history, and if they offer international positions.
- Begin with publicly available "international track" programs, but don't limit yourself. Just because a program doesn't advertise it doesn't mean they're not open—always ask and confirm.
- Many international-friendly programs don't reveal this up front but may accept unmatched international candidates during Phase II, especially if the position is still open.

In summary, general statistics provide an overview, but your approach should be highly targeted. You're not competing for thousands of spots but rather focusing on the few programs where your application, licensure timeline, and visa status align.

CONCLUSION

Pursuing pharmacy licensure and residency in the US as an internationally trained pharmacist is a complex, multiyear process involving multiple agencies, testing your perseverance alongside your qualifications. This book has guided you through this journey in phases: foundation, transition, and advancement. Ultimately, success depends on how effectively you implement what you've learned. If you're at this stage, you've likely realized that eligibility does not necessarily equate to readiness. Having the correct documents, passing exams, or completing internship hours doesn't guarantee a smooth entry into residency or long-term employment. Timing, legal considerations, state-specific planning, and immigration strategies are equally important as academic preparation.

Many capable pharmacists never finish this process, not due to lack of knowledge but because they misjudged the sequence of steps, misunderstood state board requirements, or chose a visa route that didn't align with their goals. You now have an opportunity to avoid these pitfalls.

This roadmap isn't a mere checklist; it's a strategic framework. While your specific circumstances may differ, the essential approach remains the same: Progress through each phase with clarity, minimize risks, and plan your next move before beginning.

If there's one mindset that will serve you best on this journey, it's adaptability. Regulations change. Deadlines shift. Visa policies evolve. But successful individuals don't simply react; they prepare proactively. They understand the system well enough to make informed pivots when necessary and don't assume that what worked for others will automatically work for them. Keep in mind the system might not be built for you, but success is still possible.

This journey is complicated, but you're not alone, and now you have support. Don't get overwhelmed by the steps, sequence, or requirements. I didn't create this book to make you reconsider US training. I did it to help you pursue it with clarity. Take your time, read carefully, understand each part, and then develop your plan. Remember: one step at a time. That's how I did it, and you will too.

YOUR REFLECTION MATTERS

To every reader who picked up this book, thank you!

Whether you're just beginning to explore the idea of a US pharmacy residency or you're deep in the application process, your commitment to advancing your career and crossing borders for your profession is no small feat.

This book was written with you in mind, the international pharmacist navigating a complex, competitive system with ambition and resilience. I've been where you are, and I know what it takes to succeed. This roadmap gives you not only clarity but also confidence.

Thank you for trusting me to be a part of your journey. If this guide helped you, even in a small way, I'd love to hear about it. Your success stories inspire future pharmacists worldwide.

Keep pushing. Keep learning. And don't forget you belong in the room.

Finally, if this book helped clarify things, saved you time, or helped you avoid costly mistakes, please consider leaving a review where you found it. Your feedback guides others and helps develop a documented path that often remains unseen.

Think carefully, plan accurately, and move intentionally. Your journey may be complex, but it doesn't have to be a blind one.

APPENDIX A

CHAPTER 1 TOOLS

Comparison Table of Key Features

Criteria	US PharmD Path	Bridging Program Path	Independent FPGEC Path
Eligibility	No degree or incomplete credentials or transfer foreign coursework credit	Foreign pharmacy degree + license in country of graduation	Foreign pharmacy degree + license in country of graduation
Duration	4 to 6 years (shorter for trans-fer foreign coursework credit - 2 years)	1 to 2 years	2 to 3 years
Visa Type	F-1 + OPT	F-1 + OPT	Self-managed (must already have legal US status)
Support Level	High (full academic structure)	Moderate to High (exam prep + rotations)	Low (self-guided)
Cost Range	$150K–$200K+	$40K–$80K	$15K–$30K
Residency Access	High	Medium	Low
Control Over Timeline	Medium	Medium	High

The Pros and Cons of Each Path		
Path	What You Gain	What You Sacrifice
US PharmD	Full US academic and clinical integration; high residency access; structured support	High financial cost; long duration; must meet admissions requirements
Bridging Program	Exam preparation; legal entry (F-1 visa); structured internship; potential residency access	Moderate to high cost; no residency guarantee; visa and school limitations
Independent FPGEC	Cost control; independent timeline; no need to repeat degree; flexible state choice	No built-in visa; low sup-port; complex paperwork; higher rejection risk

Pathway Comparison Summary

Step	US PharmD	Bridging Program	Independent FPGEC
Start Point	High School / Foreign Pharmacy Degree	Foreign Pharmacy Degree + License	Foreign Degree + License
Licensure Strategy	Enroll in US PharmD program	University-based bridging program	Independent FPGEC route
Visa / Legal Status	F-1 + OPT	F-1 + OPT	Self-managed / green card
Clinical Experience	Built in via curriculum	Through program rotations	Must secure US site independently
Exam Preparation	Structured by university	Structured prep for FPGEE/ TOEFL	Self-prep FPGEE/TOEFL
Internship / Rotations	University-placed internships	Moderate support (clinical sites)	Must arrange own internship

APPENDIX B

CHAPTER 2 TOOLS

US Pharmacy Residency Roadmap			
Component	Phase 1	Phase 2	Phase 3
TOEFL iBT	✓		
ECE Evaluation	✓		
FPGEE	✓		
State Selection	✓		
Internship Hours		✓	
Intern License		✓	
NAPLEX / MPJE		✓	
Residency Preparation		✓	
Residency Application (PhORCAS)			✓
OPT / Visa Status	✓	✓	✓

Strategic Checklist to Assess Your Readiness	
Readiness Checklist	Completed? (Yes/No)
I am fully aware of my visa status or have a realistic plan to obtain legal authorization for internship and residency.	
I have achieved the required TOEFL iBT scores, and they are still valid.	
I know which documents must be sent directly from my university or health authority to NABP or ECE.	
I have collected, translated, and sealed the necessary documents (transcripts, licenses, letters).	
I have started preparing for the FPGEE or have a structured study plan in place.	
I have identified the US state I will target for licensure & residency, based on realistic eligibility.	
I understand that state's internship hour requirements and pre-licensure conditions.	
I have a funding plan in place to cover exam fees, relocation, living costs, and any unpaid training phases.	
I have researched pharmacy residency programs that accept international graduates and align with my visa options.	
I have determined which year I will apply for PGY-1 residency, and my timeline aligns with that cycle.	

US Pharmacy Residency Roadmap: A Three-Phase Commitment for International Pharmacists		
Phase	Estimated Duration	Risk if Poorly Planned
Phase 1: Foundation	6–12 months	Rejected documents, delays, redoing TOEFL
Phase 2: Transition	12–18 months	Visa issues, missed internships, exam delays
Phase 3: Advancement	1–2 year	Residency rejection, employment gaps

APPENDIX C

CHAPTER 3 TOOLS

The Foundation - Phase One	
Pre-NABP Application Checklist	Completed? (Yes/No)
I have passed the TOEFL iBT with scores that meet NABP's specific section requirements.	
All supporting documents are translated, sealed, and adhere to NABP's formatting guidelines.	
I requested my transcripts and degree certificate to be sent directly from my university to ECE in sealed, signed, stamped envelopes.	
I received confirmation that ECE has completed my general evaluation report.	
I have set up my NABP e-profile and saved my NABP ID.	
My TOEFL scores and ECE general report have been sent after I created my NABP e-profile.	
I have read the FPGEC Candidate Bulletin and understand the required documents, formatting, and timeline.	
I understand that my NABP application will only be reviewed once all documents are received, and that incomplete submissions may cause delays.	

Estimated timeline (Assuming all documents are submitted correctly without any errors)	
Step	Estimated Time
TOEFL iBT Score	4–8 days ± 7 days to mail the result to NABP
ECE Report Processing	6–8 weeks ± 1 week to mail the result to NABP
NABP Application Review	8 weeks
FIC Card Delivery	Up to 4 weeks (maybe longer for international mail)
FPGEE Score Release	8–10 weeks
FPGEC Application	Valid for 2 years

Documentation Matrix

Document	Who Issues It	Use Case	Format Requirements	Who Should Send It	Submit To
TOEFL iBT Score	ETS	NABP Language Proficiency	Sent electronically via ETS after NABP profile creation	ETS directly to NABP	NABP
Degree Certificate	University	ECE Credential Evaluation	Sealed, stamped envelope	University Registrar / Mail Office	ECE
Transcript	University	ECE Credential Evaluation	Sealed, stamped envelope	University Registrar / Mail Office	ECE
ECE report	ECE	General Evaluation Report	As per ECE	ECE	NABP
Pharmacy License	Health Ministry or authorized body	FPGEC Certification	Sealed, stamped envelope	Health Ministry via official mail office	NABP
FPGEC Attestation Document	Candidate + Authorized Notary or US Embassy	Required for NABP Application	Notarized, sealed envelope	Candidate	NABP
Passport & ID Copy	Authorized Notary	NABP Identity Verification	Stamped and signed copy, optional embassy certification	Candidate (certified copy)	NABP
Photograph (passport size)	Authorized Notary	Required for NABP Application	Stamped on photo (partial), sealed envelope	Candidate (with partial stamp on photo)	NABP
Internship Completion Report	University or authorized body	State Boards / Optional Internship Credit	Certified translation recommended, sealed envelope	Candidate or authorized body	BOP

APPENDIX D

CHAPTER 4 TOOLS

Transition with Schedules and Potential Risks				
Step	What You Must Do	When to Start	Dependencies	Risk if Delayed
Secure Legal Entry (F-1/OPT/GC)	Choose your path and apply for visa	6–12 months before move	Admission, funding	Delay in entry, visa denial
Apply for Intern License	Complete application with documents	After arrival in US – at least 30 days before starting your internship	FPGEC status, SSN, US address	Can't start internship
Begin Internship	Secure preceptor and rotation	As soon as licensed or before committing to a bridging program, discuss and confirm your rotation type and site to ensure they align with your PGY-1 objectives.	Intern license issued	Residency dead-line missed
Prepare NAPLEX/MPJE	Create study plan	During internship	State approval to test	Delayed licensure
Residency Strategy	Choose programs, track OPT	Before/early internship	Program timelines	Missed PhORCAS cycle

Evaluating Visa Choices for Pharmacy Training

Status Type	Ideal For	Limitations	Can Do Internship?	Can Apply for Residency?
F-1 Student + OPT	Bridging program students	Must pay tuition, unpaid internships	✓	✓
H-1B	Licensed pharmacists	Rarely granted to interns due to high costs and restrictions	X	✓
Green Card / PR	Long-term US residents	May not apply to all	✓	✓
J-1	Research/academia roles	Prohibits direct patient care	X	X

States Selection Checklist		
Strategic Item	What to Verify	Why It Matters
Internship eligibility for international graduates	Check if the state accepts FPGEC-certified interns	Not all states accept international interns or may impose extra steps
Presence of bridging or certificate programs	See if a university in the state offers structured training under F-1	Enables legal entry and structured support
Availability of international-friendly residency programs	Review ASHP Directory or contact sites directly	Increases your match chance; some states rarely accept non-US citizens
State law exam format	MPJE, CPJE, or other? Required before or after internship?	Some exams are state-specific
Internship hour requirements	Total hours required, US only or partial credit for foreign experience	Affects duration of your training and visa timeline
Processing time for intern license	Board of Pharmacy average turnaround time	Delays here can ruin your PhORCAS timeline

States Selection Checklist		
Residency stipend eligibility	Do they pay foreign graduates? Does your visa allow payment?	Financial planning and legal compliance
Cost of living and tax burden	Housing, transportation, state income tax rates	Impacts feasibility during unpaid training periods
Long-term job market in that state	Demand for pharmacists, visa sponsorship culture	Important if planning H-1B or permanent stay
Reciprocity and license portability	Does the state allow license transfer later via NABP?	Some states (e.g., CA) are restrictive; limits future moves

APPENDIX E

CHAPTER 5 TOOLS

Preparation for Residency Application Timeline Comparison		
Step	US PharmD Graduates	International Graduates
Attend ASHP Midyear (Dec) / Residency Programs Virtual Sessions (check their website for timing)	Encouraged to attend the ASHP Residency Showcase and virtual sessions during rotations	Strongly recommended; essential for visibility, research, networking
Prepare Application Materials (Aug–Sept)	Draft CV, personal statement; request recommendation letters	Draft CV + contact US preceptors + gather documents + tailor to visa-eligible programs
Apply for PhORCAS Residency (Nov–Dec)	Before graduation	Before internship completion / licensure
Graduate from Pharmacy Program	May	Should have graduated well before May
Apply for NABP Licensure Eligibility	After completion of internship hours (already in system)	Submit after internship, or contact your university or program director
NAPLEX Approval Processing Time	2–4 weeks (usually faster)	Up to 8 weeks
License Transfer Processing Time	1 month (if needed, not typical)	Add 2 more months if transferring license across states

Residency Compensation Scenarios for International Graduates				
Funding Source	Salary Paid By	Overtime?	Healthcare Insurance?	Notes
Sponsored by Government	Government sponsor	Usually no	Depends	May not attend ASHP on paid time
Not Sponsored by Government On OPT	Residency program	Sometimes	Often yes	Confirm all terms in contract
Not Sponsored by Government H-1B (PGY-2 only)	Residency program	Sometimes	Yes	Rare for PGY-1 unless full licensure

The Advancement - Phase Three	
Pre-Application Strategy Checklist (Before PhORCAS Opens)	Completed? (Yes/No)
My internship included PGY-1 aligned rotations (e.g., internal medicine, ID, ambulatory care).	
I know when my internship will end, and it aligns with the residency calendar.	
I am tracking and preparing documentation of my internship hours for state board verification.	
I reviewed past ASHP Residency Directories and verified visa policies with programs.	
I built a list of programs that accept F-1 OPT or sponsor H-1B, are aligned with my clinical interests, and are in states that match my licensure/visa status.	
I contacted my certificate/bridging program director to ask about past residency placements.	
I got a confirmation from the university that I will be granted an OPT (if F-1) and confirmed my timeline aligns with the June–July residency start.	

The Advancement - Phase Three	
I attended ASHP Midyear (or reviewed its recordings) and connected with potential programs.	
I have a draft CV and have tailored my personal statement to target programs.	
I secured three US-based clinical preceptors who committed to writing strong recommendation letters.	
I have a plan to pass NAPLEX and MPJE before July or within ninety days of starting residency.	
I have created my PhORCAS account and reviewed its components.	
I registered for the Match and received my match code number.	

Sample Timeline Highlighting Key Dates in the Journey

Step	Target Date (2025-2027)*	What happens
Sit FPGEE	17 Oct 2025	Take the exam at Pearson VUE
Scores released	~12 Dec 2025 (8 weeks later)	Scores posted to NABP e-Profile
Apply for U.S. Visa	~22 Dec 2025 (within 10 days of score released)	Submit your visa application immediately. Allow 1–6 weeks for processing
Relocate to U.S.	~ 1 March 2026 (6 weeks visa processing)	Arrive in the U.S. before your program begins to finish paperwork
Apply for SSN	~ 10 March 2026 (within 10 days arrival)	Apply for Social Security Number using passport, visa, I-94, I-20/DS-2019 or H-1B approval. SSA mails the card to any U.S. address you list
Apply for State ID / Driving license	~ 25 March 2026 (after receiving SSN)	Get a state ID from your Department of Motor Vehicles (DMV)

Sample Timeline Highlighting Key Dates in the Journey		
Intern License Approval	~ March - early April 2026	Submit intern license application after obtaining SSN. Boards usually take 4–8 weeks to issue
Begin Bridging/ Internship	~ May - June 2026	Start your program / internship
Apply for PGY-1 Residency	~ 5 November 2026"	Apply to PGY1 residencies via PhORCAS; interviews in Jan 2027–Feb 2027 for phase I
Apply for OPT	~ February 2027	Your university's international office files your (OPT) application with USCIS on your behalf. OPT must be requested with start and end dates covering the entire residency period, usually from July 1 through PGY1's end
Complete bridging / internship hours	March – April (target) 2027	Complete the required hours ahead of PGY1 start

Sample Timeline Highlighting Key Dates in the Journey		
Participate in ASHP Match	Phase I: March 2027 Phase II: April 2027	Submit rank list and match with a PGY1 program
Apply for NAPLEX/MPJE^	April 2027 (immediately after completing your intern hours)	Register for the NAPLEX and MPJE exams through NABP and schedule your test dates promptly. University verification is required
Apply for Pharmacist Licensure (BOP)	Immediately after passing NAPLEX/MPJE^	Board processes your pharmacist license in 4–8 weeks
Receive PGY-1 Offer	~ April – May 2027	Program sends offer and onboarding packets
Confirm Pharmacist License / Pre-Employment Paperwork	~ Early June 2027	Ensure license approval, submit final HR documents, immunizations, and onboarding tasks to the residency program
Start your PGY-1 residency	~ 26 June – 1 July 2027	Start PGY1 training; orientation might be last week of June

Sample Timeline Highlighting Key Dates in the Journey		
Early commitment to PGY-2	~ Nov – Dec 2027	If you're in a PGY1 program with a PGY2 at the same institution, you can commit early to PGY2 before the Match. Always verify with the residency program director if the PGY2 position sponsors an H-1B visa or other work authorization before committing

This timeline is an illustrative example to assist you in planning your journey.

Dates are based on the 2025 NABP FPGEE exam cycle and common U.S. bridging/residency timelines. Actual dates and requirements will vary depending on: State BOP processing times, program start dates and visa appointment availability, and administrative processing for visas and background checks. Most bridging programs, such as USC GCAPP, University of Arizona Advanced Clinical Pharmacy Practice, UCSD Bridge, and MCPHS CAPPS, generally start cohorts in late spring or early summer (May–June), with some offering a fall (August–September) intake. Always verify the exact start month with the program's admissions office. Following this schedule requires strong organization, persistence, and patience, which can be tiring. Feel free to modify the timeline if you need more flexibility. it's not mandatory to follow it strictly. Create a plan that suits your needs.

REFERENCES

National Association of Boards of Pharmacy. (n.d.). *NABP. https://nabp.pharmacy*

NABP Website (for application, document submission, and licensing requirements) National Association of Boards of Pharmacy *https://nabp.pharmacy*

National Association of Boards of Pharmacy. (n.d.). FPGEC Candidate Application Bulletin. NABP. *https://read.nxtbook.com/nabp/bulletin/fpgec_bulletin/cover.html*

National Association of Boards of Pharmacy. (n.d.). *Boards of Pharmacy https://nabp.pharmacy/about/boards-of-pharmacy/*

Educational Credential Evaluators (ECE). (n.d.). *National Association of Boards of Pharmacy (NABP). https://www.ece.org/ECE/Credential-Evaluations/US-Institutions/School-and-Organization-Specific-Applications/National-Association-of-Boards-of-Pharmacy*

TOEFL iBT. Educational Testing Service. (n.d.). ETS Home. *https://www.ets.org*

Pearson VUE – FPGEE Exam Scheduling and ATT Process *https://home.pearsonvue.com/nabp*

USCIS – OPT and Visa Guidelines U.S. Citizenship and Immigration Services. *https://www.uscis.gov*

U.S. Department of Homeland Security. (n.d.). "Students and the Form I-20. Study in the States." Retrieved July 25,

2025, from *https://studyinthestates.dhs.gov/students/prepare/students-and-the-form-i-20*

Lu, C.-H., Rauf, M., Wasim, U. F., Zhang, Q., Prescott, G. M., Slazak, E. M., Desai, K. J., & Bednarczyk, E. M. (2021). "Accessibility of Postgraduate Training Program Information to Graduates from US Doctor of Pharmacy Programs Holding F-1 Visas." American Journal of Health-System Pharmacy, zxab333. *https://doi.org/10.1093/ajhp/zxab333*

Lee, J. C., Lin, P.-H., & Haaf, C. M. (2021). "Opportunities for Recruiting International Graduates of Doctor of Pharmacy Programs for Residency Training: An Academic Health Center Perspective." American Journal of Health-System Pharmacy, 78(12), 1137–1144. *https://doi.org/10.1093/ajhp/zxab136*

Badreldin, H. A., Thabit, A. K., Almangour, T. A., Al-Shareef, F., Alghamdi, M., Almetwazi, M., & Al-Dosari, B. (2021). "Pursuing Postgraduate Pharmacy Training in the United States for International Pharmacy Graduates: Approaches, Current Status, Challenges, and Future Perspectives." Journal of the American College of Clinical Pharmacy, 4(2), 224–233. *https://doi.org/10.1002/jac5.1339*

U.S. Citizenship and Immigration Services. (n.d.). Employment authorization document. Retrieved July 25, 2025, from *https://www.uscis.gov/green-card/green-card-processes-and-procedures/employment-authorization-document*

U.S. Citizenship and Immigration Services (USCIS). U.S. Citizenship and Immigration Services. (n.d.). "Optional Practical Training (OPT) for F-1 Students." Retrieved July 25, 2025, from *https://www.uscis.gov/*

working-in-the-united-states/students-and-exchange-visitors/optional-practical-training-opt-for-f-1-students

USCIS – Nonimmigrant Visa Violations Policy Manual. U.S. Citizenship and Immigration Services. (n.d.). Chapter 4—Status and Nonimmigrant Visa Violations (INA 245(c)(2) and INA 245 (c)(8)). Retrieved from *https://www.uscis.gov/policy-manual/volume-7-part-b-chapter-4*

American Society of Health-System Pharmacists (ASHP) – Residency Directory. American Society of Health-System Pharmacists. (n.d.). ASHP residency directory. Retrieved from *https://accreditation.ashp.org/directory/#/program/residency*

American College of Clinical Pharmacy (ACCP) – Residency Resources. American College of Clinical Pharmacy. (n.d.). Residency and fellowship programs. Retrieved from *https://www.accp.com/resandfel/index.aspx*

National Matching Services Inc. (NMS) – ASHP Match Stats. National Matching Services. (n.d.). ASHP match statistics. Retrieved from *https://natmatch.com/ashprmp/stats.html*

U.S. Bureau of Labor Statistics. (2024, March 29). Occupational Employment and Wages, May 2023: 29-1051 Pharmacists. Retrieved July 25, 2025, from *https://www.bls.gov/oes/2023/may/oes291051.htm*

U.S. Bureau of Labor Statistics. (2024, April 17). Pharmacists: Occupational Outlook Handbook. Retrieved July 25, 2025, from *https://www.bls.gov/ooh/healthcare/pharmacists.htm#:~:text=%24101%2C370-,The%20median%20annual%20wage%20for%20pharmacists%20was%20%24137%2C480%20in%20May,percent%20earned%20more%20than%20%24172%2C040*

University of California San Diego Health Sciences International. (n.d.). Bridge to Residency Pharmacy Program. Retrieved July 25, 2025, from *https://hsi.ucsd.edu/education/pharmacists/bridge-to-residency-pharmacy-program*

American Society of Health-System Pharmacists. (n.d.). ASHP Midyear Clinical Meeting & Exhibition. Retrieved July 25, 2025, from *https://midyear.ashp.org/*

American Society of Health-System Pharmacists. (n.d.). Residency Showcase – ASHP Midyear Clinical Meeting. Retrieved July 25, 2025, from *https://midyear.ashp.org/residency-showcase*

USC Alfred E. Mann School of Pharmacy and Pharmaceutical Sciences. (n.d.). Graduate Certificate in Advanced Pharmacy Practice (GCAPP). Retrieved July 25, 2025, from *https://mann.usc.edu/program/graduate-certificate-in-advanced-pharmacy-practice-gcapp/*

University of Southern California. (n.d.). Advanced Pharmacy Practice Graduate Certificate – USC Catalogue. Retrieved July 25, 2025, from *https://catalogue.usc.edu/preview_program.php?catoid=14&poid=20713*

American College of Clinical Pharmacy. (n.d.). Residency and Fellowship Directory. Retrieved July 25, 2025, from *https://www.accp.com/resandfel/search.aspx*

YouTube & Vimeo Academy. (2023, October 4). *International Students and U.S. Residency Application Tips [Video].* Vimeo. *https://vimeo.com/870417804/f7c1ca78d2*

American Society of Health-System Pharmacists. (n.d.). PhORCAS: Pharmacy Online Residency Centralized Application Service. Retrieved July 25, 2025, from *https://www.ashp.org/phorcas?loginreturnUrl=SSOCheckOnly*

National Matching Services Inc. (n.d.). ASHP Resident Matching Program. Retrieved July 25, 2025, from *https://natmatch.com/ashprmp/*

National Matching Services Inc. (n.d.). ASHP Match: Directory of Participating Programs. Retrieved July 25, 2025, from *https://natmatch.com/ashprmp/directory/participating-programs.html*

ACKNOWLEDGMENTS

This book stems from my challenging journey, one that many international pharmacists experience alone. When you're confronted with conflicting information, unclear systems, and silent rejections, it's easy to feel lost even before beginning. I have been through it, and I wrote this guide to offer the support and guidance I wish I'd had during my own journey.

If you're reading this book, it demonstrates your commitment to building a future in the US pharmacy industry. This roadmap is designed for you, outlining each step, challenge, and decision, not to oversimplify, but to make the journey attainable. You deserve more than guesswork; you deserve a clear, strategic approach.

To the pharmacists who asked difficult questions, challenged the system, and looked for improvements, your influence on this work is greater than you might think. To the preceptors and program directors who prioritized inclusion over ease, thank you. Your decisions have lasting effects that extend beyond a single applicant.

To my beloved family, your quiet strength and unwavering support have been my anchor. Your encouragement carried me through every page, inspiring me to keep going even in the darkest moments. Thank you for being my foundation and my hope.

Danya AlMheiri

ABOUT THE AUTHOR

Danya Almheiri is a licensed clinical pharmacist in the United States with eighteen years of comprehensive experience across four diverse healthcare systems—the United States, United Arab Emirates, United Kingdom, and Jordan. She has extensively studied, trained, and practiced within each of these regions, acquiring an in-depth understanding of pharmacy operations, regulatory frameworks, and operational challenges in both developed and emerging healthcare environments.

Dr. Almheiri completed four years of advanced postgraduate training in the United States, including a PGY-1 residency and a clinical pharmacy fellowship at Brigham and Women's Hospital, affiliated with Harvard Medical School. She also completed a PGY-2 residency in geriatric pharmacy at Providence St. Joseph Health (ElderPlace) in Oregon. Her US experience encompasses inpatient care, geriatrics, academic teaching, practice-based research, and residency mentorship.

Prior to her US training, she served as a former head of pharmacy in Abu Dhabi, where she led initiatives in pharmacy modernization, medication safety reforms, and accreditation. She spearheaded multiple pioneering projects, including perioperative medication management and the integration of technology to enhance clinical workflows and documentation, resulting in improved safety, efficiency, and accountability in care delivery.

Dr. Almheiri holds a master's degree in clinical pharmacy, international policy and practice from University College London (UCL). She is licensed to practice in Massachusetts, Ohio, Oregon, and the UAE. With firsthand knowledge of the US licensure and residency processes as an international graduate, she offers valuable insight and strategic guidance, crafted for those navigating complex career paths with clarity and purpose.

www.ingramcontent.com/pod-product-compliance
Lightning Source LLC
LaVergne TN
LVHW050935210926
848482LV00013B/623